The Best Care
for Those with the Least

An Empowering Guide to Bridge
the Socioeconomic Gap in Medical Care

The Best Care for Those with the Least

An Empowering Guide to Bridge the Socioeconomic Gap in Medical Care

Kristen Davis-Coelho, PhD

Platypus Publishing

All rights reserved.

Copyright © 2024 Kristen Davis-Coelho, PhD

No part of this book may be reproduced or transmitted in any form or by any means, electronic or mechanical, including photocopying, recording or by an information storage and retrieval system – except by a reviewer who may quote brief passages in a magazine, newspaper, or on the web – without permission in writing from the copyright holder.

The material in this book is intended for educational purposes only. No expressed or implied guarantee of the effects of the use of the recommendations can be given or liability taken. The author's experiences used as examples throughout this book are true, although some identifying details such as names and locations have been omitted to protect the privacy of the individuals referenced. The experiences of the individuals interviewed and quoted in this book have not been independently verified by the author and are conveyed here as they were reported to the author.

Interior design by Dawn Black, fiverr.com/dawnblack
Cover design by Aleksandar Novovic

Platypus Publishing

ISBN: 978-1-962133-88-3

CONTENTS

INTRODUCTION .... **VII**

PART 1: What Exactly Are We Talking About? 1

CHAPTER 1 A Story 3

CHAPTER 2 Socioeconomic Status Defined... A Few Different Ways 7

CHAPTER 3 People are Complicated: Subjective SES 19

CHAPTER 4 The Inevitable Intersectionality 27

PART 2: The Impact of Socioeconomic Status 33

CHAPTER 5 The Depressing Big View 35

CHAPTER 6 Between You and Your Patient 55

CHAPTER 7 Why? The Complex Version 67

PART 3: What Can You Do About It? Reducing the Impact
on Patient Care 89

CHAPTER 8 Common (not-so-helpful) Responses 91

CHAPTER 9 Change Is Hard... And Possible 109

CHAPTER 10 External Strategies 113

CHAPTER 11 Internal Strategies 131

CHAPTER 12 The Good Stuff 143

ACKNOWLEDGMENTS..**147**

APPENDIX A Social Determinants of Health: Patient Questionnaires 149

APPENDIX B Social Determinants of Health: Resources for Patients 150

APPENDIX C Motivational Interviewing Resources....................................151

REFERENCES 153

INTRODUCTION

How do we best serve our low socioeconomic status (SES) patients? How do we engage them and achieve positive outcomes, despite the barriers they face? How do we maintain our compassion – for both our patients and ourselves – while doing this challenging work, day after day? This book guides providers, medical teams, and administrators in exploring the answers to these questions.

The first time I presented on SES was in the late 1990s. The medical center where I had completed my pre-doctoral psychology internship asked if I would come back and present a topic for their diversity series. I suggested socioeconomic status. Most of the patients treated at the medical center were low-income and struggling, and it was clearly impacting their healthcare. Yet there had been no training, no supervision, no didactics on working with this population. Over and over, I observed well-meaning trainees and providers pathologize beliefs and behaviors that were common – and quite reasonable – for people experiencing a life of socioeconomic challenge. It struck me as a pretty big gap.

Serving vulnerable populations is my passion. I've worked as both a clinical psychologist and as an administrator in a variety of healthcare settings: inpatient, outpatient, acute, public, private, non-profit. As of the writing of this book, I serve on the faculty of the local medical school, and I treat patients at a federally qualified health center (FQHC), a community health system dedicated to treating the most marginalized members of our community. I love it. (Most days.)

In the years since I first presented on SES, I've had the opportunity to conduct training in clinics, hospitals, and academic programs on how to work more effectively with low SES patients. Attendees have shared their successes and their frustrations with me. The questions and feedback I've received most often over the years helped inform the topics that I included in this book.

My own experiences, along with those of my family members living at different points on the socioeconomic continuum, also shaped this book. I haven't always lived a financially secure life. I've personally interacted with the healthcare system both as a person with good insurance and as an uninsured person; both as a professional with a high income and as someone selling plasma to cover my bills. Look for some of those stories – not all of them flattering – on the pages that follow.

While I bring some knowledge and personal experience to the topic, I didn't want to be the only voice represented here. There's a great saying that was popularized by the disability activism movement some years ago: "Nothing about us, without us." People are the experts on their own experience. Who better to share their input and observations than the patients themselves?

So, I decided to interview other people who've struggled socioeconomically and include their perspectives in this book. I deliberately chose people who could represent a variety of experiences: some have received frequent medical care over many years; some have had much more circumscribed interactions with the healthcare system. Some have lived their whole life with financial challenges; others found themselves in that position after living a life of relative security. Some are lower middle class; some on fixed incomes; some are what you may describe as "working poor"; some have spent time unhoused.

If patient voices were going to be represented, then provider voices should be, too. I interviewed medical providers and clinical staff about their experiences working with lower SES patients; you'll find their insights, struggles, and hard-learned lessons presented here. In this case, I sought out colleagues who represented different professional experiences, different medical specialties, and different cultural and ethnic backgrounds.

Of course, labeling my interviewees as "patient" or "professional" is simplistic. All the people you'll meet on these pages have rich backgrounds, interests, opinions, and life experiences that go beyond the role they play in the healthcare system. It's also an artificial dichotomy: healthcare providers are also patients at times, and some of the patients I interviewed have worked in healthcare.

In the pages that follow, you'll find a blend of real-life stories, research findings, and practical ideas and strategies. I hope you find it enlightening, challenging, and reassuring as you do the hard work of taking care of your fellow human beings every day.

Many thanks for all you do.

PART 1:
What Exactly Are We Talking About?

CHAPTER 1
A Story

When Dr. Trudy Larson was working as an infectious disease specialist during the height of the AIDS epidemic, the first medications that came out were like a miracle. Until that point, HIV infection had been an ugly and painful death-sentence. Finally, there was hope for her patients. The protease inhibitors weren't perfect; in fact, they were a pain-in-the-butt. They had horrible side effects; they had to be kept refrigerated; they had to be taken with food five or six times per day. But they were lifesaving. Care for her patients with HIV/AIDS changed dramatically almost overnight. And then one day a patient asked a question Dr. Larson wasn't expecting:

"What if I don't have a refrigerator?"

Dr. Larson had worked with patients who were struggling financially her whole career. She was used to conversations about not being able to afford medication or co-pays. But this was different. "An 'aha-moment' – a major one," is how she describes it now. Not only did she discover that some of her patients didn't have refrigerators, but patients she had worked with for years began admitting that they didn't have enough food to take with the medicine. "It was so hard for them to tell me this," Dr. Larson recalls.

While some of these patients were unhoused, most were working low-pay jobs or on fixed incomes and living in weekly motels – with microwaves, but no refrigerators. She was aware *in theory* of the challenges her patients faced, but the experience opened Dr. Larson's eyes to what daily life was like for them. "Holy cow," she says, reflecting on her medical training, "I didn't ever learn that I had to ask people if they had refrigerators or if they had enough food!"

The healthcare professionals I know – and I've known many over my career – are dedicated, compassionate people who are committed to doing their best for every patient. But we don't know what we don't know. These days, the medical field is doing a better job recognizing the impact of social determinants of health (SDoH) – those things that impact patients' health that aren't "medical" in the traditional sense, such as access to quality food, a safe environment, the resources to afford care, and social and economic policy. The work that researchers, academics, and policymakers are doing in this area has increased our awareness of how broken the healthcare system is for marginalized patients, including those living at the lower end of the socioeconomic scale.

But what to do about it? Even the most conscientious healthcare professional is facing barriers of their own: seeing patients back-to-back all day; squeezing more patients into shorter and shorter timeframes; trying to complete all the screening tools and visit requirements that have nothing to do with why the patient is there. Not to mention clicking endlessly through the EMR, which – let's be honest – does not exactly add joy and fulfillment to your day.

Even some of the patients I interviewed for this book expressed awareness and empathy for the challenges their care teams face. As one patient, Chad J., put it, "They might get at their wits' end with being able to provide the best care for each individual patient, because there's only so much time." He noted that these demands make it harder for the care team to "set the experience for the patient up for success."

The challenges patients and providers face are many, large, and systemic. We're more aware of them now, but your typical provider, medical assistant, nurse, or administrator doesn't have the time – or frankly, the power – to make the kind of systemic changes needed to fix our healthcare system on a large scale.

Despite not having that power, who is held responsible for patient outcomes? You are. A1C levels, hospital readmissions, viral load, depression scores, hypertension control, BMI, preventive screenings, ER turnaround times, birth weights, surgical outcomes… Clinical outcome and quality measures have become an everyday part of practice. And real consequences are tied to meeting them.

Not only are external forces expecting you to impact patient outcomes, but I suspect you hold yourself responsible as well. People who are drawn to work in the medical field tend to be hyper-responsible folks to begin with. You're here to help people, to make a difference, to fix problems. Fixing problems is the whole reason for your professional existence: if you can't solve the problem your patient is presenting, what are you doing there?

So how do you fix the fact that your patient doesn't have a refrigerator? Or paid time off to go see the specialist? Or enough money to fill their prescriptions consistently?

This is a vicious combination:

Awareness of a critical problem + being held responsible for solving it + having zero ability to do so.

Responsibility with no control = powerlessness.

Awareness without tools = burnout.

Healthcare professionals need effective and practical tools to help the patient sitting in front of them today. I'm not talking about medical interventions. I'm a clinical psychologist; you won't catch me advising you on medical treatment. But I do have expertise in changing perspectives, changing behaviors, and changing how we practice. My goal is to help you examine your assumptions about socioeconomic status in fresh ways; to engage more effectively with your patients; to make your interventions more accessible to the patients who need them most. Hopefully you'll come away feeling a little inspired, a little more empowered, and recognize the difference you're making in people's lives every day.

Let's dive in.

CHAPTER 2
Socioeconomic Status Defined... A Few Different Ways

It's rewarding to know that you helped somebody that might have fallen through the cracks.

- Dr. Faith Whittier

Defining Socioeconomic Status

Most of us have a basic understanding of what we mean when we refer to socioeconomic status... It's how much money someone has, right?

Actually, socioeconomic status is a surprisingly complex concept. If you dig into this area, you'll find rigorous and passionate debate about how it should be defined. Beliefs about what it is and how it should be measured have changed dramatically over time. Though there are some measures that are used more commonly in research than others, coming up with a universal definition has been elusive, to say the least. Some argue that it's impossible. The complexity of this discussion – though fascinating – is way outside my area of expertise and way outside the purpose of this book. My goal is to give you enough information to frame – or reframe – your conceptualization of socioeconomic status as it applies to your practice. Here we go.

SES can be defined by composite measure or by proxy measure. Composite measures include more than one data point or piece of information that's then combined into an overall result. When it comes to SES, there are a few primary factors that are almost always included as part of the composite measure. As you read the examples below, try to identify those primary factors:

Jessica is a writer with a master's degree who rents a room and works odd jobs to support herself while she finishes her novel; Jerry barely finished high school but wrote a bestseller and made lucrative movie deals for each of his subsequent three books. Chan's family has a significant amount of wealth and he's paid a ridiculously high salary for the position he holds in his uncle's company... though he didn't graduate and doesn't do any real work. Marcus has a bachelor's degree, works hard as the case manager in a group home, and makes $52,000 per year; Monique has a bachelor's degree, works hard as the financial controller for a large multi-site medical practice, and makes $112,000 per year. After attending medical school, completing his residency, and passing his Boards, Manuel works as a family physician and makes $225,000 per year. After earning her high school diploma, completing an apprenticeship, and passing the test for her contractor license, Maria works as an electrician and makes $66,000 per year.

As you probably figured out, the three primary factors typically used in composite measures of SES are education, income, and occupation. For many individuals, these three factors are congruent and easy to classify, as in the last couple of examples above. But you can also see from the earlier examples that a difference in one of these factors appears to change a person's SES dramatically. The possible combinations are many and varied.

The examples also highlight two different aspects of socioeconomic status, which I think of as Resources vs. Respect. You can also think of them as breaking the term "socio-economic status" into economic status and social status. SES invariably implies an economic element that includes practical, tangible resources such as money and transportation. But "status" also implies one's position in the social hierarchy, including how much someone is esteemed or valued by the dominant social structure, how much power they have, and their access to social capital.

Usually, these two aspects go hand in hand. But not always. Jessica in the above examples would likely have higher "respect" or social status than monetary resources. The "struggling artist" archetype, if you will. And if she writes a few highly popular and influential bestsellers but donates all the profits to charity, her social status may increase while her economic status may not.

The examples also demonstrate the heterogeneity of the group who would be classified as low SES based on the three factors: They might have a low educational attainment, or a low income, or an "unskilled" or "semi-skilled" occupation… but they don't necessarily have all three. Some folks in this category may fit neatly into the stereotypical image of a "lower class" person. But there's a wide range of people deemed "low SES," and many won't fit the usual stereotypes.

Rather than a composite measure, some research uses individual proxy measures. Using a proxy measure means you're measuring one factor that's strongly correlated with the thing you actually want to study. Socioeconomic status is a complex concept, and one indicator is easier to gather than three (or more), particularly if you're doing large-scale population studies or relying on publicly available information. So, some of the research relies on one factor as a reasonable "stand in," or proxy, for SES.

The three factors above – income, education, and occupation – are each also the most common proxy measures; some studies use earned income alone, some use educational attainment alone, and – fewer, but they do exist – use occupation. Other factors that have been suggested as proxies include wealth, defined as accumulated assets; access to resources; and location of residence or – more specifically – the median value of owner-occupied housing in their location. Each of these proxy measures has its own advantages and limitations.

Whether you're using a composite measure or a proxy measure to capture SES, it's based on objective data points. But as we'll see shortly, objective data isn't the only – or even the most important – information when it comes to the patient sitting in front of you. However, what's clear is the relationship of SES to health outcomes. Speaking generally, the higher the income, educational attainment, or occupational status, the longer one lives.

SES Classifications

In everyday conversation, many informal labels for different socioeconomic levels exist. We might talk about the poor, the working poor, or one that I heard recently: the "educated poor." People may refer to someone as "solidly middle class." We might say someone is blue-collar, white-collar, rich, or uber-wealthy.

Of course, the problem with these informal labels is that there's so much room for interpretation. I may assume that you and I are talking about the same thing, but we may in fact mean something very different. I'll never forget the reaction of one of my family members when they overheard a physician-couple refer to themselves as middle-class; with a large house, high income, regular vacations, and more vehicles than adults to drive them, they certainly didn't meet this person's conceptualization of middle-class. This person considered themselves – with a much lower income and a career in skilled labor – to be a prototypical example of the middle-class.

Fortunately, standardized classification systems exist in which key factors related to SES are combined and weighted to yield a specific SES level. In fact, many standardized scales exist. Before we look at the overall SES classifications, let's take a moment to look at how each of the individual factors are defined.

Education

You've probably filled out demographic questionnaires that ask about educational attainment. These fall into two different types: Continuous measures or categorical measures. Continuous measures simply ask for the highest year of school completed and the person responds by writing down a numerical value: 11, or 14, or 18, etc. Categorical measures break it down into – you guessed it – categories. These might look like the following:

- Less than high school diploma
- High school diploma or equivalent
- Some college
- Four-year degree
- Post-graduate degree

Sometimes it's broken down further, including a category for a technical or trade certification, an associate degree, or separating post-graduate study into master's degree or PhD/medical degree. In some research targeting specific populations, investigators choose categories that make the most sense for that population. For example, we'll look at a study later in which the impact of SES, race and gender was being examined in a population with an overall low level of educational attainment. For that study, participants were divided into two categories: Those with less than a high school diploma were categorized as "lower education" and those with a high school diploma and above were categorized as "higher education."

Income

Likewise, income is typically broken out into several categories. On demographic questions, the categories may look something like:

- Less than $50,000/year
- 51,000-100,000/year

- 101,000-250,000/year
- $250,000-$500,000/year
- Over $500,000/year

In terms of income labels, these five categories are often used:

- Poor
- Lower-middle class
- Middle class
- Upper-middle class
- Wealthy

Note that the income amounts listed above and the labels listed above don't actually correspond to each other. Income categorization is based on many factors, not the least of which is where you live. An annual income of $70,000 dollars is a very different thing in rural North Dakota than it is in New York City.

When you're focused on a lower income population, the categories within poverty and lower middle class may be divided more finely. In this case, the income levels are often based on the Federal Poverty Level, or FPL. FPL is a measure of income established by the Department of Health and Human Services each year. For 2024, the Federal Poverty Level is equal to or less than an annual income of:

- $15,060 for an individual
- $20,440 for a family of two
- $25,820 for a family of three
- $30,000 for a family of four
- And so on, up to $52,720 for a family of eight

Eligibility for various benefit programs, tax credits, etc., are often determined by a person's income relative to the Federal Poverty Level, such as being below 150% of the FPL, or between 100 and 400% of the FPL. Community health centers called Federally Qualified Health Centers (FQHCs) use FPL to determine whether a patient qualifies for a sliding fee scale and what their fees are for different medical services. Researchers who are focused on this low-income group may use similar divisions to determine the income aspect of socioeconomic status.

In 2022, the most recent year we have complete data for, the official poverty rate in the U.S. was 11.5%. This translated to 37.9 million people living below the Federal Poverty Level. [1] Put another way, more than one out of every ten people in the U.S. was attempting to eat, have housing, and support their family within the incomes described above.

Occupation

If you do an internet search for "occupational categories," you'll find a wide variety of classification systems. Some of these systems have more of a conceptual basis; some are practical; some are statistical. The number of categories varies widely; for example, one of the most commonly used systems in the US is the Standard Occupational Classification system, or SOC. The SOC identifies 867 individual occupations. These detailed occupations are then grouped into 459 broad occupations, 98 minor groups, and 23 major groups. [2]

On the other end of the continuum, the most basic way to categorize occupation is within three "labor" categories. The categories are based on the amount of training and requirements for the position. The categories are:

- Unskilled: These are often entry-level positions that don't require specialized knowledge or education, and most often involve some form of on-the-job training. Examples include delivery driver, janitorial worker, food prep positions, or agricultural worker.

- Semi-skilled: These jobs require some specialized skills and experience, but rarely require an advanced degree or complex technical knowledge. Examples include security guard, flight attendant, retail sales, health care aide, or truck driver.

- Skilled: These occupations require specialized knowledge and specific training to execute physical or mental tasks. This skill level exists in both "blue collar" and "white collar" professions. Skilled positions could include an accountant, an electrician, or a physician.

Now let's be clear: These labels are controversial, and for good reason. All jobs require skills, and jobs classified as "unskilled" are some of the most physically or mentally demanding. Imagine the server in a busy 24-hour diner working the "bar rush" overnight shift: Within a span of three hours – right after the bars close – they serve 50 tables full of inebriated customers. These folks show up in waves and may not be the most clear, organized, or considerate in their demands. The server must strategize the pace and timing of greeting, taking drink orders, delivering beverages, taking food orders, delivering food, checking back, and delivering checks to each of those tables.

All within the unpredictable timing of new tables being seated, people being ready to leave, and food being ready to serve. And all with a pleasant demeanor and a smile. Having worked this job during college, I can tell you the level of multi-tasking and shifting priorities under immense time-pressure is equivalent to that of a busy ER on a Saturday night. No, lives aren't on the line. But a big chunk of your income is controlled by the people you're serving.

Overall SES

As you can see, there are a wide variety of ways to measure the different factors that go into overall SES. Efforts have been made to standardize these, and guidelines have been suggested about the best ways to do so. These efforts are helpful, because they ensure that the results of different studies based on SES are comparing apples-to-apples.

So far, we've been talking about individual SES: one person's educational attainment, their personal income, and their current occupation. But there are broader ways of examining SES, too. "Family SES" includes those same factors for all adult members of the household, as well as considering the combined income, savings, and material resources and assets of the household. A professional with high educational attainment and a solid income may be upper middle-class as an individual. If they're the solo earner in a family with six kids, have few assets and a lot of debt, their family SES is going to be much lower.

"Neighborhood" or "community SES" attempts to capture the average SES of a defined region, such as a census tract, block-group, or zip code. What is the median income in that area, the percentage of people with different levels of education, the types of occupations represented? This is an important consideration because some health outcomes can be more closely related to community SES than the individual SES of a person who lives there.

All of the above examples and classifications are based on objective data. A person's annual income, the highest education they obtained, and their current job are all facts that exist and can be verified. To conduct valid research, objective information is key. But when it comes to our patients, it's probably not as important as another way of viewing socioeconomic status: Subjective SES, or subjective social status (SSS).

Subjective SES is just what it sounds like: A person's perception of their socioeconomic status. How we perceive and experience our SES relative to others may or may not be congruent with the objective facts. And in fact, a fascinating and robust body of research has demonstrated that subjective social status is more strongly associated with a person's physical health and psychological well-being than their objective SES.[3-9] So, what are some of the factors that can influence a person's subjective assessment? We'll explore that in the next chapter.

Reflection

At the end of each chapter, I've included some questions for you to consider and reflect on. These questions are simply offered as a way to interact with the concepts, ideas, or recommendations discussed in that chapter. Feel free to ponder them, write your responses, or save them to review at another time. If you find them useful, I'd be happy to send you a complete set of reflection questions in a format you can use and share. My contact information is included at the end of the book; feel free to reach out to me directly.

1) What labels have you used informally to refer to people at different points on the socioeconomic continuum?

2) Consider the three primary measures for SES: income, education, and occupation. How do these three factors interact in your own current circumstances? How have they interacted at different points in your life?

3) Using the income categories for the Federal Poverty Level, how much could a family of four spend on housing each month? How does this compare to the average cost of housing in your area?

CHAPTER 3
People are Complicated: Subjective SES

I always thought, How the heck? You have nothing, but you still give.

- Dr Trudy Larson

Transient vs Chronic

Josh is a young medical student. He works at a local restaurant as a waiter; he also works a side gig driving people, food, groceries and whatever else anyone needs. He's exhausted all the time and is embarrassed about the amount of credit card debt he's accumulated. He hasn't been spending frivolously. He barely makes enough money to cover his bills, so when an unexpected expense comes up, he has to use his credit cards. Like last month when his old car died on the side of the road. He's worried about how many student loans he's taking to cover tuition, and he has an anxiety attack every semester when he signs another set of loan documents. He deals with the stress *by reminding himself that it's temporary: he's working toward a goal that will include a good job and a good income. He looks forward to finally having some financial breathing room and daydreams about how he's going to spend his money.*

Fast forward 10 years: Josh is a young physician in a group practice. He makes six figures, is slowly paying off his student loan debt, and is looking forward to buying his first house. He knows he has the option to work at one of the agencies in town that qualify for student loan forgiveness, but he really likes the practice he's in, so he's staying there for now. Josh is being smart with his money. He only uses his credit cards when he knows he can pay them off at the end of the month, and he's already saving for retirement. He's far from rich, but he's comfortable and has enough extra income to do a lot of the fun stuff he could only dream about during med school and residency.

Jack is a young waiter. He works at a local restaurant doing the dinner shift six nights a week. When he's not at the restaurant, he works a side gig driving people, food, groceries, and whatever else anyone needs. He's exhausted all the time, but he's good at his job and already talked to his manager about training to be a bartender so he can make better tips. Jack is embarrassed about the credit card debt he's accumulated covering unexpected expenses, like last month when his old car died on the side of the road. Lately, when a bill shows up, he finds himself fighting an anxiety attack. He's hopeful he can move up in the service industry and find some financial breathing room.

Fast forward 10 years: Jack is the lead bartender at a nice hotel and gets all the prime shifts. During the day he drives people, food, groceries, and whatever else anyone needs. His pay has gone up over the last 10 years and his regulars tip him well, but the cost of living has outpaced his income. His credit card debt is out of control. He works to pay it down, but then another unexpected expense comes and all the progress he's made is wiped out. The panic he used to feel when he paid his bills has turned into a tightness in his chest that never goes away. He has no idea how to climb out of the hole. He knows he'll be living this way the rest of his life, unless he hits a financial crisis and ends up homeless.

Our subjective experience of our socioeconomic status is hugely influenced by whether our current situation is transient or chronic. Though it's hard in both situations, experiencing a low SES is very different when we have a reasonable expectation that it's temporary.

Stable vs Unstable

Small business owners, professional artists, people working on commission, or someone relying on unreliable child support may enjoy a comfortable income… some of the time. Maybe. Unpredictably. The stability of our income or occupation has a big influence on our subjective perception of our socioeconomic status. A friend who's a professional in the tech field had a surprising number of layoffs early in his career. Over and over, he came home to tell his wife he'd been laid off and they needed to cut expenses and not make any plans until he found another position. Later, he realized the pattern: He'd take a position in a new start-up and as soon as the business was ready to go public or be acquired, the employees with the highest incomes would be let go. Why? To improve the cost/profit ratio on paper. Even though the family was easily middle class while he was employed, the sense that they couldn't rely on that income and at any moment it could be taken away had an unsettling impact on their subjective social status.

External Indicators

Our SES is reflected in what we present to the world. Our clothes, shoes, haircut, car, and home tell the world a story about what we do and how we do. But sometimes our objective SES and these external indicators are incongruent.

When I was young, my family lived in a big house in a nice rural/suburban area. My dad was a professional with a college degree and my stepmom worked in a semi-skilled position. But with four kids and various habits and hobbies that took our discretionary income and my parents' attention, we didn't look middle-class.

We shopped at second-hand stores – before it was trendy – and each kid got two pairs of pants, five shirts, and one pair of shoes for the school year. At the beginning of the year the pants were too big, and by the end of the year they were threadbare and too short. And always about five years out of style. There were weeks at a time that I don't remember brushing my hair or taking a bath. We had a junk-pile of old cars in the front yard, my siblings and I ran around unsupervised, and the whole neighborhood could hear my mom hollering at us down the quiet suburban street. Yep. We were *that* family. Even though on paper our SES would have been solidly middle class: Professional parent with a college degree, two incomes, big house, assets... we were perceived as the "poor" family in the neighborhood, and I felt conspicuously "low class" compared to my peers.

In contrast, I worked with a patient many years ago who always came to his appointment in a nice suit and dress shoes. It was several weeks into therapy before he acknowledged he was on the verge of homelessness. He had bought the suit after receiving a small inheritance, and he liked how the world treated him when he appeared to be a successful professional. Now the money was gone. His financial situation was growing more and more dire, but that reality was hidden behind an expensive tie.

Social support

Having a solid support system and other types of resources can buffer our perception of our SES. A low-income, working single parent who has no social support, no childcare resources, and no one to help in a financial pinch would experience their socioeconomic status very differently than a low-income, single working parent with a neighbor who watches the kids, a handy friend who comes over to fix things, and a grandpa who happily loans money when things are a little too tight. Having access to emotional, practical, and financial support when needed can change our assessment of our own status in life.

Generational

My late husband grew up proudly blue-collar. His father's family came from an agricultural background and his dad was a mechanic. People worked with their hands in the fields or in the shops for many generations. They weren't just proud. There was an undercurrent of bias against well-off and highly educated people in their household; his father would joke derisively, "Those doctors don't even know how to change their own tire!"

Then my husband went to college. Married someone with a PhD. Got a job that involved an office and a desk and more mental effort than physical... And suddenly he belonged to the group that he had been raised to scoff at.

Our SES isn't just objective facts about our life; it becomes part of our identity. When our status is significantly different – either higher or lower – than what's been typical in our family across generations, this can have a profound impact on our subjective perception. Imagine two individuals living very similar lifestyles: They have a decent place to live, a modest but steady income, a reliable used car, and if they pay attention to their budget, they can save up to take a trip or buy something frivolous. Now imagine that one of them comes from a family with "old money." They grew up in private school, buying expensive clothes on a whim, trips to exotic locations, and spending the summer at the family vacation home. They took this lifestyle for granted; not because they were spoiled, but because for them – and for all the people around them – it was just normal.

Imagine that the other person grew up in poverty. The family repeatedly lost their housing and had to live in their car; they got the free lunch at school but never knew if there was going to be enough food for dinner; they stayed with random neighbors while their parents worked odd shifts or traveled to find work. A modest, stable lifestyle makes the first person feel poor; the second feels like they won the jackpot. We can't help but compare ourselves – explicitly or implicitly – to where we came from.

Comparison group

Similar to external indicators and generational influences, who we use as our comparison group can have a profound influence on how we perceive and how we feel about our socioeconomic position. If your friends, neighbors, or co-workers live a higher SES lifestyle than you, it's easy to feel like you're missing out. Their home is nicer, they have "extras" you can't afford, and you scroll enviously through pictures of their latest vacation on social media. On the other hand, if the people you hang out with on a regular basis have less than you, that influences your subjective social status in a very different way.

For our patients who are lower SES, the comparison group doesn't have to be people they know in real life. It's everywhere: in the movies, social media, walking down the street, in the doctor's office. The awareness of how you're struggling, while others apparently are not, is acute and constant.

Reflection

1) How would you characterize your socioeconomic status while you were growing up?

2) What factors influenced your perception and experience of your SES then?

3) How would you characterize your SES currently?

4) What do you expect it to be 10 years from now?

5) If you expect it to be different, why? To what do you attribute the change?

6) Do you think others would perceive your SES the same as you do? If not, why?

CHAPTER 4
The Inevitable Intersectionality

I think that all of it is kind of intertwined. That's why it's so difficult... I think SES might be at the center.

- Dr. Jose Cucalon Calderon

We can't talk about socioeconomic status without acknowledging its interaction with other factors that impact the healthcare a person receives: Race, ethnicity, geographic location, gender, age, sexual orientation, disability, primary language, gender identity, body size… Intersectionality plays a significant role in this space. Along with SES, each of these factors is connected to the care people access (or can't) and the care they receive (or don't).

Are healthcare outcomes the result of poverty, or race, or where someone lives? The answer to that question determines how the discrepancy should be addressed. Good research has been attempting to tease out the independent and combined influence of these factors for many years. The results are not simple; for example, the relative influence of SES versus race differs by gender, geographic location, how you measure health status and outcome, the disease process being studied, which racial/ethnic groups you include, and how SES is defined. When you add in gender, geographic location and other factors, the results become even more complex.

A classic example is a study published in 1993 by Guralnik, et al.[10] They examined the interaction of socioeconomic status, race and gender on health status. For this study, SES was captured by the proxy measure of educational level, and health status was measured both as total life expectancy and as active life expectancy (which was defined as life expectancy without significant physical limitations). The study participants all came from the same geographic area, which at the time had manufacturing as its primary economy and an overall low level of education. For our purposes I'll just highlight the results related to active life expectancy and the interactions between educational attainment, gender, and race.

The first analysis was based on educational level. Among Black study participants, men with higher education had an additional 2.9 years of active life expectancy over Black participants with lower education levels, while women with higher education levels had an additional 3.9 years. For White study participants, men with higher education levels had an additional 2.4 years, and for women 2.8 years. The next analysis divided participants first by race, and then looked at gender and educational attainment. They found that White men with lower education lived 0.9 years longer than Black men with lower education; White men with higher education lived 0.4 years longer than Black men with higher education. However, for women, they found that White women with lower education lived 0.4 years less than Black women with lower education, and White women with higher education lived 1.5 years less than Black women with higher education.

Some of these findings are counter-intuitive, and even this small sampling of the study's results demonstrates the complexity of the interactions between different factors. It also highlights the importance of knowing how different factors are defined. In this study, which was conducted in an area with an overall low level of educational attainment, higher and lower education was defined by whether someone had graduated from high school.

In the three decades since that classic examination, many studies have attempted to tease out the relative influence of different sociodemographic factors on health outcomes. For an excellent survey of the research on these interactions, I'd recommend Donald Barr's book, *Health Disparities in the United States: Social Class, Race, Ethnicity, and the Social Determinants of Health (3rd edition)*.[11]

As Dr. Jose Cucalon Calderon, a pediatrician working in a teaching hospital and community family medicine clinic, indicated in the quote at the beginning of this chapter, many people working with disenfranchised populations have come to view SES as the core driver of healthcare disparities for those groups. While there is, of course, evidence that other demographic factors play an independent and often powerful role, the idea that SES holds a significant amount of the variability is a compelling one.

When it comes to the patient sitting in front of you, sometimes the combined effect of belonging to more than one marginalized group is obvious. A patient who is both poor and speaks a primary language other than English is going to have far more challenges navigating the health care system and implementing their care plan than someone with only one of these barriers. And the more of these factors a person identifies with, the harder it becomes. The challenges don't just multiply. They increase exponentially.

The more marginalized groups your patient identifies with, the more likely it is that you won't have all of them in common. You may share a primary language and ethnic background, but you grew up middle-income in the suburbs and they live in an impoverished urban center. And what if you and your patient do share a lower SES background? How does that impact your relationship with your patient and the care you provide them? We'll take a look at that question a little later, but just a teaser: While this confers some benefits, it's not without its own risks.

All the providers I interviewed highlighted the importance of making a connection with their patients. The more marginalized the patient is, the more important that connection is. While this connection may be easier if you share specific socio-demographics, acknowledging the similarities and differences opens the door for a relationship.

Dr. Cucalon Calderon talked about his first experience practicing in a small, rural, economically depressed town deep in the southern United States. Growing up in a completely different culture in Ecuador, raised in an educated family, and speaking

English as a second language, there were so many differences between him and his patients, Dr Cucalon Calderon says, "I felt like a Martian." And he didn't just feel like one. The patients viewed him as a Martian, too. But by being open to his patients' experiences and approaching them in a spirit of respect and curiosity, he was able to develop a connection with them.

Dr. Faith Whittier, a Black American OB/GYN who has spent her career working with low-income patients in community health centers, spoke about the benefits of having the same racial or cultural background as your patients. When she and a patient don't share a common background, she says, "meeting that person where they are and figuring out how we can connect," is still critical. "I think that crosses all intersections if you can make that connection," she says, "Because you can find different ways to make it. It may be we have a cultural connection, it may be that I understand poverty too, or just your experience… A common human experience you can align on."

Reflection

1. As you read each of the below examples, imagine the specific healthcare challenges each of these individuals might face:

    a. An American Indian woman who lives in an isolated rural area

    b. An American Indian woman who lives in poverty in an isolated rural area

    c. An American Indian woman with a physical disability who lives in poverty in an isolated rural area

    d. An elderly man with a visual impairment who lives in an urban center

    e. An elderly man with a visual impairment who lives in an urban center and speaks limited English

    f. An elderly transgender man with a visual impairment who lives in an urban center and speaks limited English

2. Visualize some of your patients who embody different sociodemographic factors that could impact their healthcare. As you think of them, consider:

    a. Which potential impacts do you recognize most easily?

    b. Which do you notice, but minimize?

    c. Which do you have a blind spot for?

PART 2:
The Impact of Socioeconomic Status

CHAPTER 5
The Depressing Big View

It's a culture shock.

- CHAD J.

So far, we've talked about what socioeconomic status is, how it's defined, the difference between objective and subjective SES, and the intersection with other diversities. What about the interaction of socioeconomic status and healthcare? Let's dive into that next.

The impact that a patient's socioeconomic status has on their health outcomes and the healthcare they receive is a long and – depending on your mood – either depressing or infuriating story. Maybe both. The not-so-surprising end to the story? Lower SES patients have poorer health and often receive subpar care.

Before we jump into the impact of SES at the individual provider level, let me touch briefly on the interaction of SES and population-level health outcomes. Obviously, these are related, but overall health outcomes are not really the focus of this book; that's more in the realm of policymakers and epidemiologists than individual providers. But the findings are striking and provide some "macro" context before our discussion of the "micro" impacts at the level of provider and patient.

Fifty years of research across several countries, different measures of SES, and different measures of health can be summarized as follows: At a population level, the lower your income, your educational attainment, and/or your occupational status, the worse your overall health, the higher your likelihood of experiencing illness and disability, and the lower your life expectancy. This does not appear to be a "threshold" model; that is, it's not that once you get below a particular SES threshold you see these health impacts. Rather, the impacts appear to exist on a continuum from highest to lowest SES. As the World Health Organization website summarizes it: "In countries at all levels of income, health and illness follow a social gradient: the lower the socioeconomic position, the worse the health." [12]

The reasons are complex: In the United States, many are related to the fundamental structure of the healthcare system; the history of how access to care has been tied to geography; the intersectionality of SES and other marginalized groups; the way our financial systems and the business of healthcare is designed. It's also related to many factors that aren't directly connected to healthcare, such as the chronic nature of stress for people at the lower end of the SES continuum, poor air quality in lower income urban settings, targeted predatory marketing of junk food and nicotine products, lack of safe communities, and so on. A thorough discussion is outside the scope of this book, as are the very cool ways researchers have teased out the impact of different aspects of SES and other variables. If you're interested in a detailed examination, once again I recommend the excellent book *Health Disparities in the United States: Social class, race, ethnicity, and the social determinants of health*, by Donald A. Barr. [11]

It's helpful to stay cognizant of the fact that the patient sitting in front of you lives within the system that contributes to those poor outcomes. In some ways, when you're working with a patient to address a specific medical issue, you're also fighting against these larger forces. It's an uphill battle for both you and your patient. Below, I'll highlight a few of those forces that come up commonly in discussions with patients and providers.

The payer system

Many of the patients I interviewed were quick to point out that they have great medical providers and are grateful for their public health benefits. But the barriers that exist for them in navigating the healthcare system often feel insurmountable.

"It's beyond something that is manageable for somebody that's on top of their life, let alone somebody who is having multiple issues," says Lona S., a patient I interviewed who was completing a bridge housing program as part of her journey to secure permanent, stable housing. Lona was talking about attempting to navigate what she refers to as "The Medicare/Medicaid Money Matrix." She shared that she had already been on Medicaid based on her income level, but then was unexpectedly signed up for Medicare when she qualified for disability benefits.

Though she initially assumed having both insurance programs would be a good thing, Lona shared stories of spending hours on the phone trying to get information about lab work or medication that was being denied coverage, only to be told she had to call the other benefit office and wait on hold again. She was told she couldn't make an appointment at the local Social Security office; she simply had to show up and wait and hope that the person who had the right information was available that day. Which they often weren't. When she was finally able to get questions answered, different people or departments would give her conflicting information about what she needed to do, essentially paralyzing her from moving forward. Lona reported that despite her current life struggles, she is fairly well educated and organized. "I can't imagine somebody that's having way more cognitive issues, or pain issues, or homeless issues, or no-transportation issues, or 'do I have clean clothes?' issues," she said, "I don't even have those issues and it's very, very difficult for me."

Another resident in the same bridge housing program, Feather C., described trying to get treatment for a chronic issue: "I needed to see a podiatrist. You can look on your phone, and there's an endless amount of podiatrists. I have to go to [a city 450 miles away] to see a podiatrist. There's nobody here that will take the Medicaid." Feather reported that because there were no local providers, Medicaid would cover the transportation to the appointment with a certain amount of advanced notice. So, she scheduled the appointment with the podiatrist as far in advance as she had been instructed, and then scheduled the transportation. A couple of days before the appointment, Medicaid contacted her and said they actually needed more advanced notice than they had initially told her. Feather called the podiatrist, rescheduled the appointment, and booked transportation again according to the new instructions. Once again, shortly before the scheduled appointment, Feather was contacted and told they needed more advanced notice... After the third time, Feather cancelled the appointment and decided to postpone addressing the issue altogether, despite the pain and impact on her mobility. She said she appreciates her benefits: "Medicaid covers things, they've never really declined much on me, but you have to do so much leg work yourself, and in the meantime, you need to work."

Anyone who's dealt with a chronic or acute medical issue themselves or with someone they love has navigated the complexity of the healthcare system: referrals, what's covered and what isn't, which providers you can see, where and how to access needed care, tracking appointments and follow-ups. These challenges are magnified for those dealing with Medicare or Medicaid because of the limited access and added levels of bureaucracy.

The experience of limited choice for people with socioeconomic challenges was a common theme in my conversations with patients. Chad talked about the difference between his previous life as the director of a successful art gallery at Lake Tahoe and now, "I'm not living in Incline off the Lake like I was for 20 years. And I don't have the income that I used to have... I went off the deep end with drugs and so I lost all that." Chad described the dramatic difference between having good private insurance plus the money to pay for any treatment he wanted or needed, and then finding himself in the public health system, "It's a culture shock." While he expressed gratitude for the community health center where he receives good care, he doesn't have the choices he used to. Chad described a specific test he had received in the past for his chronic medical condition, but that his current provider doesn't utilize. Before, if he felt strongly about needing the test, he would have simply paid out-of-pocket. He no longer has this option. "I'm in a different boat now," he says.

Another lack of choice that low SES patients experience is when providers make decisions about treatment or interventions without discussing them first. Anecdotally, patients who are on Medicaid report this experience more often than patients with private insurance. Jenna W. shared an example when her son – who was covered by Medicaid at the time – visited the dentist. The staff told her that her son would get sealants applied, and she could choose whether it happened at that visit or the following one. They did this without discussing it as a recommendation, or even explaining what sealants were. Jenna described how the "choice" she was offered – do it now or do it next time – didn't feel like any choice at all: "I was like, 'Uh, there's a third option here or maybe even fourth, and I'll research it and decide if I want to do it at all.' Felt like a total fail at informed decision making on their part."

Likewise, Feather described her experience consulting with an orthopedist for a knee problem: "Because I'm on Medicaid… there's only one guy in town. And he wanted to schedule surgery before we did the MRI… He was pushing the operation. And because there's only one – I mean, there's numerous in town, but because he's the only one that takes Medicaid, he's got a lock on it. I can't go get a second opinion unless it's out of my own pocket."

The patients I spoke to didn't necessarily hold the providers or care teams responsible for all these challenges; they're aware of the complexity of the system and the fact that care teams themselves face similar challenges trying to navigate it. When Feather needed cancer treatment and the oncologist was reviewing treatment options,

> *The doctor told me, 'Well, this is what I'd like to do, but Medicaid won't cover it.' I'm like, 'Too much money?' And he's like, 'Well no, actually it's cheaper.' He said it's cheaper, it's more effective, but he's like, 'Who knows [why it isn't covered]?' A lot of it is lobbying… there's a lot of money behind the scenes. An awful lot of money. And I just feel like when you're on the lower end, you're a number.*

The gap

A few weeks ago, I found myself in line at an urgent care clinic. The man ahead of me – who looked like he felt as awful as I did – was at the front desk checking in. He gave the staff his insurance card and then started politely asking questions: How much was his co-pay? What would that include? What if he needed follow-up? He was clearly trying to decide if he could afford to pay for the visit or if he needed to leave without being seen. The front desk clerk didn't bother hiding her impatience: she was abrupt, she interrupted him, her facial expression and body language radiated annoyance. As he stood there vacillating, I stepped forward and offered to pay his co-pay for the urgent care visit. He hesitated; I said it would be a gift to me if he allowed me to pay; he politely declined.

This was the first time I'd offered to pay someone's co-pay for a medical visit. I've paid for people's prescription co-pays at the pharmacy a few times; you can hear the stress in someone's voice when they realize the cost for their medication is more than they can afford. If the cost isn't extravagant, I'm happy to make sure they can leave that day with the medicine they need. Of course, there are risks involved: My offer could be rejected, the person could be offended, or I may endure a bit of social awkwardness during the exchange. We'll also talk in a later section about the dangers of "over-helping." But overall, these experiences have been positive for both me and the other person, and it allows me to feel like I'm contributing to the challenges of the world in a small, practical way.

Back to the urgent care clinic: After we were both checked in and seated in the waiting room, the man approached me to introduce himself and thank me for my offer. He explained that he could afford the co-pay today, but that he also had an appointment with his doctor about another issue later that week, and he only had the money to pay for one of them. He had been trying to decide which need was more critical. He was frustrated that he had to take a day off work to come to urgent care – his first day missing work in over a year.

This is one example of a "gap" that people experience: They have private insurance through their job but can't afford to use it. Sometimes this is because of a high deductible, co-insurance, or co-pay, sometimes because they have chronic conditions or multiple issues that require frequent care. Sometimes it's simply because all their income is accounted for by their living expenses, and an urgent care co-pay is an "extra" they can't afford.

Here's another common gap: between private insurance and public benefits. Ivy Spadone, a PA-C (certified physician assistant) who has spent her career working with disenfranchised patients and now also teaches in a PA program, recalled a patient she treated who had HIV along with other chronic conditions. To receive medical care, he had to quit his current job to take one that paid less. Yes, paid *less*. The higher paying job didn't offer health insurance. He made too much money to qualify for benefits that cover treatment for low-income patients living with HIV, but not enough money to afford his own insurance. Even though he had the opportunity to move upward in his vocation and income – and his overall life stability – the gap during which he would not qualify for public benefits and not be able to afford private insurance would be life-threatening. He took the lower paying job.

These gaps are frequently on the minds of both patients and providers. As Feather put it,

> *I'm literally scared because I've got to make more money to get on my feet again. But when you leave the Medicaid all of a sudden you're at the hands of insurance companies and that's expensive… It's not just losing the Medicaid, I'll be losing any food benefits. There's no real safety net when you're going up, you know? When you're falling down there's a safety net, it's up to you to do the work to get into the net. But when you leave, it's not a tier thing. It's like, today you made 28 thousand dollars and 42 cents, you qualify for all of this. Tomorrow you make 29 thousand and you get nothing.*

Food

The next time you're at your favorite grocery store, do a little experiment: Look at the price of apples. Nothing special, just nice, big apples. Do a little math: How much is it for four? Next, look at the strawberries. How much for a half-pound container? Add those two costs together.

Now consider the "value menu" or "dollar menu" at your favorite fast-food place. How many of those cheap burgers can you get for the same price as four apples and a container of strawberries? Imagine that your fridge is empty, and you only have a few dollars left to buy food. Whatever you buy is all you'll have to eat until you get paid at the end of the month. Which choice makes more sense?

Of course, this assumes you can even access a grocery store that carries fresh fruit. You've probably heard the term "food desert": A geographic area where nutritious food is expensive or unavailable. These food deserts are usually found in low-income, historically marginalized communities and they're associated with high rates of chronic disease.

Dr. Steven Shane, a pediatrician and obesity medicine specialist who has worked in acute, emergency, and outpatient settings, points out, "Getting your food at the 7-11, little bodegas, it's all what you're exposed to and what's at hand." He points out that both transportation and money are barriers for people to have any option for purchasing groceries other than at a convenience store. If the public transportation system is inadequate, "Some people have to take two hours to get somewhere you could drive in ten minutes."

Similarly, Dr. Cucalon Calderon talks about how food access and food insecurity was his biggest "aha moment" when he began working in a low-income community:

> I was delivering a lot of lifestyle change recommendations, and they had a significant amount of children dealing with obesity and some of them with health complications. And one of the easy answers – it became like an eye-opening moment – 'Well, the only thing I can buy is chicken nuggets.' 'Okay, how about the big bags of broccoli?' 'Uh uh. The chicken nuggets last longer. They last longer, they don't get spoiled, I can freeze them in batches.' Now I know that there are food deserts… at the time I had no idea. I was seeing it, but I had no idea that's what it was.

In that community, Dr. Cucalon Calderon recalls, "To get good vegetables, you had to drive 45 minutes."

As long as we're doing experiments, try this one: Drive to a lower SES neighborhood in your community, go to the local convenience store, and attempt to grocery shop. Not just for a few things you want or need, but a complete set of groceries to feed a family. Besides being more expensive than you would find at a larger supermarket, trying to eat a reasonably healthy and varied diet from what you can get there is quite a challenge.

As Dr. Shane highlights, "You can teach people until you're blue in the face about what they should do – and I think a lot of people know what they should do to stay healthy – but to be able to deploy the plan and execute it is a whole different situation for them." And beyond those individual challenges, Dr. Shane points out that some of the contributions to health discrepancies are even more insidious. "One thing a lot of people don't think about," he says, "is the predatory marketing toward lower socioeconomic status individuals and people of color. That's a biggie."

Environment

There are a whole range of environmental factors that can impact people's health outcomes. These include transportation, housing affordability, housing quality, neighborhood characteristics, amount of green space, and building density, just to name a few. A complete review of these factors would fill a whole book, so we'll just look at a small sample: Housing, built environment, and transportation.

Housing

I did therapy for several years with a kid who lived with his family of four in a tiny studio apartment. It was cramped, to say the least. The small living space served as family room, bedrooms, and dining room all at the same time. There was no privacy except the single bathroom, there was no space for a dining table, and there certainly wasn't enough room for any form of physical activity. The kids had no quiet place to study and the parents had few opportunities for adult conversation. Their neighborhood wasn't the safest, so free time was spent indoors. The parents were doing the best they could to maintain a strong family: They took the bus across town and back every week to attend therapy sessions, and never missed a medical appointment for the kids. But the stress of so much "togetherness" in their tiny living space, especially as the kids grew into teenagers, took a toll on all of them.

The family I worked with was fortunate, however. None of them had significant medical issues. Many families living in this situation include family members with chronic or acute medical conditions: A child with asthma, a parent with diabetes, a grandparent with mobility issues and dependent on oxygen. Imagine attempting to manage all the prescriptions and medical equipment for multiple people sharing one small bathroom, in addition to all the regular bathroom supplies and grooming equipment.

A lot of attention is being paid to housing affordability these days, and rightly so; it affects almost everyone, not just those in a low socioeconomic position. However, as rough as it is for everyone, the cost of housing has a disproportionate impact on people with a very low income. The U.S. Census Bureau tracks a multitude of data, including the "housing cost ratio," which is defined as the percentage of household income that goes toward rent or mortgage plus utilities. In 2021, U.S. Census data shows that for renters living in the lowest income quintile, the median housing cost ratio was 62.7%. [13]

This statistic means that half of the lowest-income renters paid *more* than 62.7% of their total income for rent and utilities each month. Pull out your calculator and do some quick math: Type in your annual income and multiply it by .627. Now divide that by 12. How does that number compare to your current monthly housing and utility costs? What kind of impact would it have on your ability to pay for medical care if this much of your income went toward having a roof over your head and electricity?

In addition to the challenges of inadequate living space and cost, there's the issue of quality. Lower income communities often deal with aging infrastructure and poor construction. Older homes and buildings are more likely to have issues with black mold, lack of air conditioning or heat, lead paint, asbestos, and unsafe drinking water.

Built environment

The impacts aren't only at the level of individual housing. The larger physical environment also plays a role. A 2018 study by Besser and colleagues examined the impact of the built environment on the health of the people living there. Built environment included building density and resources for walking around the neighborhood. You can get an idea of this by imagining spaces where the buildings are crowded together and the sidewalks, paths, or crosswalks are small, damaged, or non-existent. They found that worse quality of the built environment was associated with more rapid cognitive decline of the residents, particularly in African Americans. [14] Other studies have demonstrated the impact on health outcomes from a variety of objective neighborhood characteristics, as well as resident perception of neighborhood safety, cohesion, deprivation, and aesthetic quality. [15-17]

Transportation

Transportation is a huge barrier for many patients. I was speaking with a patient the other day about his challenges following up consistently with his specialty care. He explained that he didn't have a car, and he lived on the outskirts of town where the bus only comes every two hours. He had to take two transfers to get into town. To get from his house to his appointment – which would take about 45 minutes by car – he was getting a multi-hour scenic bus tour of the city. Both directions. His roommate was willing to drive him to appointments, but the roommate only received his shift schedule two weeks in advance – a common experience for people who do shift-work. This meant that if the patient wanted a ride, he couldn't schedule appointments further ahead than two weeks. Getting a specialty appointment less than two weeks in advance was, of course, nearly impossible.

Transportation can be an even larger problem for people living in a rural area. They often spend two or three hours driving to where their care is, and then two or three hours driving back home. A simple medical appointment becomes an entire day event.

As researchers have discovered, environmental impacts on health for lower socioeconomic community members can range from the micro – mold levels in older housing contributing to asthma severity – to the macro – building density and lack of safe outdoor spaces. Dr. Shane talked about what he learned from families he worked with:

> *I got a really good education doing the healthy living program. You just learn what people's barriers are trying to implement the things that they learn and what they know they should do to try to be healthier. The transportation issues, parents working one or two jobs each, the kids are fending for themselves at home, playing videogames, they can't go outside because it's not safe. You hear about, 'Oh, there was someone shot in the park last week.'*

Another type of "environment" also plays a key role in health: The social environment. We'll talk about one aspect of the social environment next – the impact of significant social stressors on health.

ACEs

You've probably heard of ACEs, another factor that significantly impacts health but isn't traditionally medical in nature. ACE stands for Adverse Childhood Experience. These involve the social environment and events that are experienced during childhood; specifically, ACE refers to stressful experiences that people may be exposed to as they're growing up. ACE scales include items that assess for:

- Physical, sexual, or verbal abuse
- Physical or emotional neglect
- Parental separation or divorce
- Living with a household member struggling with mental illness
- Living with a household member who abuses drugs or alcohol
- Living with a household member who attempted or committed suicide
- A household member who went to prison
- Witnessing a parent being abused

Twenty-five years of research has yielded robust findings about the impact of these childhood experiences on our physiology and their link to future mental and physical health outcomes. Just a few highlights: The higher someone's ACE score in childhood, the more likely they are to develop cancer, diabetes, heart disease and stroke as an adult. Higher ACE scores are associated with a variety of chronic health conditions, increased risky health behaviors, and early death. According to the CDC, at least five of the top ten leading causes of death are associated with ACEs. In terms of mental health, people with higher ACE scores are more likely to struggle with depression, bipolar disorder, substance misuse, and suicide. [18]

So why include a section on ACEs in a book about socioeconomic status? Research demonstrates that children living within a low SES are more than twice as likely as their higher SES peers to have had three or more adverse experiences. While this is a fact, I worry that mentioning it risks reinforcing stereotypes about people who live in a lower SES. We all know these experiences – substance use, divorce, emotional or physical abuse – aren't limited to one geographic, racial, ethnic, or socioeconomic group. Stress and trauma can impact us all.

However, there is also a potentially cyclic nature to SES and ACEs. As noted above, the lower the SES, the higher likelihood of adverse experiences. But the reverse is also true: The more adverse experiences one has in childhood, the higher likelihood they will have a low SES in adulthood. It can become a tragic multi-generational cycle.

It's also worth noting that the ACEs scales don't capture all potential childhood stressors. In particular, they don't do a good job capturing community-level trauma and stress. These scales don't typically ask about exposure to crime or community violence, the stress of chronic under- or unemployment, or the impact of discrimination.

Despite the significant impact adverse childhood experiences have on health, few medical practices ask the families of pediatric patients about these experiences or ask their adult patients about past experiences. Doing so could give the medical team key information about preventative care, as much as asking about a family history of heart disease or cancer.

Often, patients don't volunteer this information either, even if it's happening in real time. Dr. Shane tells the story of a young man he was seeing for treatment of obesity. They had been making good progress on the young man's health habits when suddenly all the forward movement started backsliding. Dr. Shane recalls, "It was one of those situations where I didn't ask in any way, 'What's different?'" He found out later from another member of the care team that the patient's older brother had died from an overdose.

Keeping these potential stressors in mind – whether you assess them formally or simply inquire about stressful life experiences – will give you key health information about your patients. Asking about them also clearly tells the patient that these life events are an important aspect of their health, and opens the conversation for the patient to bring it up when it's relevant.

Two patients

Early in my career, part of my job involved providing consultation on the medical floors in the local Level II trauma center. Most of my consultations were in the pediatric intensive care unit. I worked with children and teenagers in the ICU who had terminal illnesses or traumatic injuries, conducting psychological evaluations or meeting with the kids in their hospital room for psychotherapy. One year, within the span of several months, I was asked to work with two different kids who came into the ICU with traumatic spinal cord injuries, resulting in quadriplegia.

The parents of these two children suddenly had a lot in common. What was different, though, was the amount of occupational and financial resources they brought to the situation. As the days moved forward, their initial shock evolved into wrapping their heads around life with a child who was permanently paralyzed from the neck down. This is when the impact of their socioeconomic positions became clear.

The first set of parents were at the hospital all day every day. They spent time on the phone with their employers, delegating their tasks and applying for family medical leave. Within a few days of the accident, as reality started to sink in, they talked about moving their son's bedroom to the ground-level floor of their home. They began making plans to put a ramp in at the front entrance and modify the downstairs bathroom to be wheelchair accessible. Managing these practical aspects seemed to help them get back some small sense of control.

The second set of parents took turns at the hospital while they continued to work intermittent shifts at their jobs. Without paid leave and living paycheck-to-paycheck, if they didn't work, they couldn't pay their bills. I overheard them tensely trying to figure out which job was more likely to fire them if they asked for "too much" time off to be with their son. Within a few days of the accident, as reality started to sink in, they realized they'd have to move. Because they rented, they couldn't renovate their home to be wheelchair accessible. With the help of the social worker, they located an accessible apartment they could afford, but it was in another part of town. Their children would have to transfer to new schools.

Both sets of parents were devastated and overwhelmed; no level of resources or social position can change that. But the limited resources of the second family added layer after layer of stress and complexity to an already excruciating situation.

Throughout this chapter, most of the socioeconomic impacts we've been talking about are the day-to-day kind. But these challenges are magnified when you're dealing with a medical crisis, whether that's a parent with a terminal illness, a critical diagnosis for your spouse, or a life-changing injury to your child.

Reflection

1. Reflect on the systemic barriers described in this chapter – the payer system, coverage gaps, food, housing, transportation, environment, and ACEs. Of these:

    a. Which ones do you think are having the largest impact on your patients?

    b. Which ones do they share with you?

    c. Which ones do you suspect are impacting your patients, but you never hear about it from them?

CHAPTER 6
Between You and Your Patient

It's hard – implicit bias, we all have it. I think you just have to be constantly conscientious of tone of voice, facial expression, how I sit… Lots of times they'll thank you for not being judgmental. When someone does that, it makes you feel good.

— Dr. Steven Shane

If you're reading this book, then I assume you are a compassionate, dedicated person who works hard for the best outcome for all patients. Maybe you even work harder for the ones with the least resources. Despite that, we must acknowledge that the subpar care lower SES patients receive doesn't just happen at a population level; it happens on an individual basis between the care team and patients every day. Some of the reasons are ones you can probably predict, some are subtle and surprising, but let me just say: I do not for a minute believe that it's because you don't care. It's hard to take care of the medical needs of people who have so many other needs as well. But with a few small changes, you have more power than you realize. More on that later.

Implicit Bias and Cultural Competence

You've probably heard of implicit bias; it's been a large part of the discourse on disparities and discrimination in recent years. While there is no universal scientific definition of implicit bias, it refers to preferences, beliefs, and stereotypes that we hold and that are applied automatically, unintentionally, and without our awareness. For a simplistic example: Imagine a kindergarten teacher. What image first popped into your head? If you're like most people, it was a woman.

These implicit beliefs may even be in opposition to our consciously held and expressed values. For example, someone may consciously believe that men and women are equally capable of succeeding in any professional position, but they may also hold an implicit belief that men make better leaders. Without realizing it, this person may spend more time informally mentoring the men in their department than the women.

If you'd like to explore the topic of implicit bias further, a good place to start is Harvard's website, Outsmarting Implicit Bias: A Project at Harvard University. [19] They provide learning modules and an overview of cognitive biases and findings based on Implicit Association Tests. If you'd also like to check out some articles and studies that are critical of the science behind the implicit bias concept, check out the repository on the Open Science Framework. [20]

The concept of cultural competence is also worth mentioning. Although it's traditionally been applied to racial and ethnic cultural differences – and it's not without its limitations – it's worth considering SES through this lens. One common way of conceptualizing cultural competence is three-fold: 1) Awareness of your own personal beliefs, attitudes, values, and biases, 2) Awareness and knowledge of the worldview of individuals and groups from the relevant culture, and 3) Utilization of culturally appropriate strategies and interventions. One of the limitations of this model is it risks missing the heterogeneity within the group, and that's certainly true for SES.

Cultural humility is a concept that some prefer over the idea of cultural competence; it acknowledges that you can't know everything about every culture or group. Cultural humility involves an openness to learning about others and the impact of culture and identity, awareness of one's own culture and potential biases, and lifelong learning. As Dr. Cucalon Calderon suggested, "By being open to learn about them, you are going to be able to – or at least I was able to – navigate a lot of the difficulties." As applied to socioeconomic diversity, this book aims to help you become more culturally competent, or culturally humble, or perhaps both.

It's also worth mentioning that most providers come out of their training programs with some experience working with low socioeconomic status patients. Low-cost clinics and safety net hospitals are often the setting for clerkships, training hours, and rotations. Having this experience can give clinicians the impression that they have specific competence in treating low-income patients. But the fact is, exposure alone doesn't lead to competence. If you saw cardiac patients as part of your training in a primary care setting, does that make you competent to provide cardiac care? You'd want specific training and education with that patient population before you considered yourself competent in that area. Both experience and education are required.

What If You Come From a Similar Background?

It's only natural that our reactions in working with patients from diverse socioeconomic backgrounds are influenced by our own background and experiences. Someone who has experienced poverty themselves is going to bring a different perspective than someone from a more privileged background. If you share a common background or sociodemographic status with your patients, it's bound to influence your interaction.

Is socioeconomic status unique?

Socioeconomic status is both similar to and different from other sociodemographic factors that influence the medical care people receive. I think about these factors as varying across three dimensions: How consistent the factor is across time; how intentionally malleable it is; and how obvious your status is to the patient sitting in front of you.

It's easy to identify factors that remain consistent across time. For example, if you're Black now, you also grew up as a Black person, and you can be pretty sure you'll be Black in the future. If you share the same race with your patients, there's some element – or at least an assumption – of common experience there.

Other sociodemographic factors are malleable. You may belong to different groups at different points in your life. For example, you may have grown up on a farm in a rural agricultural community, but now live in a high-rise apartment in a large metropolis. Or vice versa. You may have lived the first half of your life as a large-bodied person and now are slender. Or vice versa.

Most relevant to the current discussion is whether your patients are aware that you belong to a particular sociodemographic group. In most cases, there are certain factors that are immediately obvious to others, such as race, gender, weight, or physical disability. But there are plenty that aren't visible, and socioeconomic status – or more specifically, the socioeconomic status you grew up in – is one of them. Think about this: You may have grown up in the same public housing project as the low-income patient sitting with you talking about their diabetes. But unless you were neighbors, how would they know that?

There is one way that I believe socioeconomic status is truly unique: SES is the only sociodemographic factor that is inherently changed by the very nature of your professional role. Just the fact of having attended medical school, PA school, nursing school, or a radiology tech program, and now working as a professional, changes your socioeconomic status. Education and occupation, as you'll recall, are two of the primary factors for determining SES. A nurse who grew up low SES is now automatically in a different status based on their education and occupation, as well as their income. Likewise – and more so – for a medical provider. Having a professional education and working in the medical field inherently moves you out of a low SES category.

Think about the other sociodemographic factors you might share with a patient. None of them are changed by the very nature of your role in healthcare. This makes SES unique. As Dr. Whitter points out, "Education can't change race, right? And so race tends to be a bond that just exists. Period. It doesn't matter what kind of educational background you have." In contrast, your role as a medical professional means that you and your patients no longer share the demographic connection of being low SES, even if that was your history.

But what if you're still living in a lower socioeconomic status? There are plenty of people reading this book who – despite being part of the medical team – are still struggling in a low-income bracket. Unfortunately, some occupations on the care team do not automatically put people in the middle class: CNAs, MAs, and med techs in different specialties, just to name a few. Though these roles require training and skill, the monetary value placed on them is often not enough to significantly impact the income part of the SES equation. For these folks, their socioeconomic challenges are much more likely to be similar to the low-income patients they're taking care of: living paycheck-to-paycheck, worrying about their housing, one crisis away from a financial disaster. As we talk about socioeconomic status, it's important to recognize that some of our colleagues may be just as affected as our patients.

Potential benefits

If you come from a lower-SES background, there are potential benefits for the relationship with your patients and the care you provide them. The primary one is your awareness of the challenges they face. If you understand having to navigate a crappy public transportation system, or deciding which bills you can pay and which ones you have to skip, or being judged because of your clothing or your zip code, this direct experience is invaluable.

Demonstrating your first-hand knowledge of these barriers can also help build a connection with your patients. As both patients and providers point out, this connection is critical for building trust and increasing engagement in care. You don't have to disclose your history directly to demonstrate this understanding, either. Asking the right questions in a matter-of-fact way or validating their perspective with details that only someone who's "been there" would know tells patients that you "get it."

This direct knowledge also helps reduce some trial-and-error when a treatment plan isn't working, or the patient is struggling with adherence. You're in a better position to hypothesize what the barriers might be and check those out with the patient early in the process.

Potential pitfalls

However, don't assume that having a similar background to your patients guarantees you're going to be more effective with that population. In my experience, there are a few potential pitfalls in working with patients from the same background.

If we're from the same demographic group, it's easy to conflate our experiences, beliefs, and history with that of our patients. If they're presenting in a certain way or struggling with their care, you may assume you know what's going on based on your own experiences. We need to remind ourselves that there are a huge variety of individual differences even for people who live in the same community, zip code, or on the same street. It's critical to take an open, curious approach and check our assumptions.

Another potential pitfall: We work with a low SES population and come from a low SES background ourselves; therefore, we identify with our patients and assume they'll automatically identify with us and feel a connection. But it doesn't matter if we're still living down the street from them, buried in credit card debt and student loans; our patients will not necessarily see us as one of their own. The "higher" we are on the continuum of medical education, the more salient this disconnect becomes.

Interestingly, patients in an extremely high socioeconomic status (the top 1-3%) may also not see us as being able to relate to their lives in a direct and practical way. Even if we grew up within this demographic or belong to it currently, unless the patient knows that, they will also perceive a status difference and assume that we can't relate to their particular challenges and barriers. (Check yourself: Did you just have an automatic reaction to the idea that the very rich may also have healthcare barriers?)

Another potential pitfall is that because we see ourselves as similar to our patients, we feel less of a power differential between us and them. But the moment we put on that white coat (either literally or figuratively) we're automatically in a different SES class than those patients. The risk is that we may underestimate the impact of the power differential on our patients' interactions with us.

Finally, some professionals may just want to move on from the socioeconomic struggles of their past. They no longer want to carry that identity; they want to "fit in" with their new professional peers; they want to distance themselves from the past. The risk is that this desire impacts their interactions with low SES patients; they may be more distant, more business-like, less willing to acknowledge or talk about the patient's life circumstances that are affecting their care. There also may be an implicit bias of, "I made it out, why can't you?"

Impact on patient care

As we reviewed in an earlier chapter, SES has significant impacts on health outcomes at a population level, and the reasons for this are ridiculously complex; start down this path and you'll find yourself in some fascinating - and infinitely deep - rabbit holes. But what about the interactions that happen on a day-to-day basis between healthcare professionals and patients?

Although far more research has been conducted on the impact of patient race and ethnicity on these interactions, there's a fair bit that is focused specifically on SES. We'll review some of those findings below. A disclaimer first: This isn't designed to be a comprehensive review of the topic; there may be newer or better research out there at this point. If you're aware of some, feel free to email me – I'd love to hear from you. This section is designed to be a taste, a sampling, to give you an idea of how patient SES can affect provider behavior.

The first big impact we see is on the healthcare provider's perception of the patient. Studies have demonstrated that lower SES patients are perceived as less intelligent, having less self-control, less rational, less likely to be compliant with medication, less likely to follow-up, and less likely to have significant job demands or responsibility to care for family members; they're also perceived as having lower levels of social support, poorer health, and a worse prognosis. [21,22] SES also affects clinical assessment: Lower SES patients' pain was perceived to be less intense, was more likely to be attributed to psychological factors, and was perceived as less credible. [23]

SES also affects the type and timing of diagnosis and referral. For example, lower SES patients have later referral to pediatric neurosurgery, [24] later referral for chronic kidney disease, [25,26] and are less likely to be referred to Phase I cancer clinical trials. [27]

Treatment recommendations are also impacted by patient SES when all other factors are equal. Research has demonstrated that patient SES impacts recommendations for the form of contraception, [28] elective sterilization, [29] acute non-specific low back pain, [30] major depression, [31] comfort care versus resuscitation at peri-viability, [32] diabetes technology for youth, [33] management of diabetic neuropathy [34], cardiac procedural care [35] and intervention for prostate cancer. [36]

"Sure," you might be thinking, "A provider has to consider the patient's means, resources, and insurance type when they're deciding on referrals and treatment options. That's just reality." Of course, that's true. Providers frequently struggle with having to balance what they know is best practice with what is realistic for a specific patient's circumstance; it's a source of daily stress for providers trying to give the best care to all their patients.

However, it's important to note a few things. First, a number of studies that find differences only include patients across all

SES levels who have private insurance, in order to minimize the impact of payer type on provider decision-making. Second, most of the studies examining provider perception utilize a randomized experimental design with either video or written clinical vignettes. In these vignettes, the only thing that varies is the SES of the patient; everything else is identical. Finally, some results simply can't be rationalized. For example, with identical clinical presentation and history, and even using a standardized assessment tool that's designed to negate provider idiosyncrasies and biases, assessment of cardiac risk was still impacted solely by patient SES. [37]

Reflection

1) In what ways does your own socioeconomic background support your ability to relate to your patients? In what ways does it make it more challenging?

2) Which of the research findings cited above were a surprise to you? Which ones weren't? Why?

CHAPTER 7
Why? The Complex Version

People are cut off by themselves and by the systems that don't see them because they have fallen through so many cracks.

- DARLENE K.

So why these differences? In this chapter, we're not talking about structural oppression embedded in the fundamental nature of our entire healthcare system, or about the rare provider whose bias against low SES patients is overt and unapologetic. We're also not going to attribute the differences to implicit bias and call it a day. We'll be exploring the "why" that impacts caring, dedicated team members in their day-to-day moments with patients. And by talking about that "why," we'll be able to talk about strategies to address it.

Formal training versus Narratives

Learning comes through a variety of modalities. We learn from what our professors say, from the books and articles we read, from our clinical supervision and case review, and certainly from our own professional experiences. One powerful way humans learn is through stories. Politicians and advertisers know this well; if you have the choice to present a whole series of facts or one impactful story, choose the story every time. People are more likely to remember it and be swayed by it.

The same holds true during our training experiences. Your instructor, your textbooks, your curriculum can say all the right things about working with socioeconomically diverse patients, yet one story shared by a respected mentor will always have more power. In a classic article from the mental health field, Dr. Phoebe Kazdin Schnitzer posited that much of our learning about working with low-income families happens via narratives – repeated stories, explanations, and attributions – handed down informally across time from supervisor to supervisee or colleague to colleague. [38] From my observations over the years, the same informal learning path applies in the medical field.

Dr. Schnitzer suggested that these narratives fall into three different themes. Let's consider how these themes might present themselves in medical settings:

"They don't come in"

You see a patient, they have a newly developing or existing medical issue, you make recommendations and a treatment plan, schedule a follow-up... and never see them again.

Or you see them three years later when the untreated issue has progressed into serious consequences. Or you never see them at all until they present in the ER.

When providers talk about productivity in the context of lower income patients, the rate of no-shows and cancellations is always brought up. This belief – that low SES patients no-show and late-cancel more often than middle and high SES patients – is so entrenched that this question is rarely examined objectively. At a population health level, when rates of preventable illness or death are discussed, the blame is often placed on the patients for not seeking the care they need. These discussions often have a "what can we do about it?" shrug-of-the-shoulders subtext.

"They're so disorganized"

Patients consistently arriving late for appointments, no-showing, not getting critical lab work done, dragging the kids along into the exam room, or forgetting your instructions. This is another implicit narrative that makes its way into conversations about low SES patients. Often the subtext here is around assumed cognitive or intellectual deficits, and an inability to manage their own life. Later in the book, we'll talk about the Self-Serving Bias, which has special relevance to this narrative.

"They don't care"

Perhaps the most damaging of the narratives that exist around lower SES patients, I believe this one is borne of provider burnout as much as anything else. When a patient doesn't do what they need to do – or when a perceived group of similar patients don't – this is often the final fallback narrative. The same issue has come up repeatedly, a needed action still hasn't happened, and finally this narrative comes out. "I've made it as easy for them as I possibly can; it's not that hard; if they cared about their health at all they'd just get their lab work done/check their blood sugar/take their medication/eat a little healthier/follow-up with the specialist…

This narrative is also applied to parents as related to their child's mental or physical health. When follow-up doesn't happen as timely as the provider expects, or interventions at home aren't implemented consistently, or a parent isn't perceived as taking a medical issue seriously, with low SES families there's an assumption that the parent simply doesn't care about or prioritize the child's needs.

Interestingly, narratives don't just exist on the professional side of the patient/professional relationship. Patients also have common narratives that they apply to their providers and healthcare agencies. Like the professionals' narratives, these are passed informally from person to person. For patients who are struggling financially, these narratives often center around agencies or providers not caring or not understanding what it's like to be in their position.

Sometimes this narrative applies to a specific provider or entity, e.g., "X hospital doesn't care about their patients, they just want to make money." Sometimes it's about a specific level of care. For example, several patients I interviewed indicated that they experience the most socioeconomic bias when they're in the ER. Lona stated it directly, "The ERs are a nightmare... It's just a condescending, rude attitude. If you're going into healthcare, don't you think you should like people?" Sometimes these patient narratives encompass the whole healthcare system rather than specific people or entities. Darlene K., a professional who's had periods of her life when medical issues have significantly impacted her socioeconomic position, asserted, "It gets reinforced every day by family members, by neighbors, by friends, 'Oh yeah, my doctor doesn't get it either.'"

My conversations with teaching providers give me cause for hope. For example, PA Spadone has incorporated specific learning experiences for her students around working with low SES patients. Every year, she invites a panel of patients who were previously unhoused to come and present to the students. In PA Spadone's courses, she specifically talks about serving low SES patients and individuals experiencing homelessness, "I always tell them, 'These are my peeps, these are my people. I love serving the underserved.'" This language, plus hearing the experiences of low SES patients directly during a training program, is a powerful opportunity for students to come into the field with a wholly different narrative than the negative ones described above.

Population data versus individual data

Imagine a lower SES patient sitting in front of you. Their labs indicate a few preventable health risks on the horizon. You begin talking with them about how to incorporate more physical activity and healthier food choices into their life.

Sounds like good preventive medicine, right? But think: Did you ask them specific questions about their current diet and exercise patterns? Or did you jump into recommendations?

Base rate and population data are important in medicine. We can't assess every possible issue with every patient, and knowing the prevalence of different health behaviors and medical conditions tells us where to focus our attention. The fact that lower SES patients – as a population – have lower levels of physical activity and lower quality diets is well-known and well-validated; you're probably aware of this finding without even consciously thinking about it. The problem occurs when population data overrides individual data. In the literature, this is called "statistical discrimination," and it often shows up in two forms.

In one form, we neglect to validate that the base rate information applies to this specific patient. In the above example, we don't ask the patient about their own physical activity and food habits before we start making lifestyle recommendations. We simply assume that the population data applies to them.

In the second version of statistical discrimination, we ignore, discount, or minimize information the patient is telling us because it contradicts population data. If the above patient had told you during previous visits that they're a distance runner and a vegetarian, but the salience of their low SES overrides that information and you start talking to them about developing healthy habits, that's statistical discrimination.

In the absence of contrary information, or when the information you have is ambiguous, relying on population data makes sense. But the individual patient sitting in front of you should always be given more weight.

Communication: The care team side

What is the most critical part of an effective clinical encounter? Knowledge? Skill? Time? I'd argue that there's another factor that is even more foundational. When it works well, visits are quicker, more effective, and more rewarding for both patient and medical personnel. Without it, patients can't get their needs met, a provider has no idea where to even start their assessment, and the risk of complications and tragic outcomes skyrockets. And yet, this is the piece that most often goes wrong. It's the root cause of many poor outcomes, malpractice suits, and patients lost to care. What is this magical factor that has so much power for good or for evil? Communication.

Take a moment and reflect on the patients that make you feel most positive in your role. Now think of a few that you feel less effective with or even dread seeing. I'm guessing that how well or how poorly the communication goes between you and those patients is at least part of the reason for that difference.

I like to divide these communication influences into ones that live primarily on the provider side of the equation, and those that live on the patient side. Of course, it's impossible to separate them completely, and we'll look at the interaction a little later. For now, let's start with the communication factors that lie primarily on the care team side.

Medicalized language

Medical school teaches a new language. It makes sense that specialized knowledge comes with specialized vocabulary, shorthand, abbreviations, and a way of communicating information. Unlike language learning that's designed to be used with the group being served – think learning a foreign language to go and teach in that country, or to open a business there – this language is a language by providers, for providers, between providers. Isn't it a bit odd that the language learned is one that isn't spoken or understood by the people it's meant to help?

Medical jargon is one of the main barriers in communication in a healthcare setting. I don't use the term "jargon" pejoratively. Basically, I'm referring to those words, phrases, labels, and abbreviations that healthcare workers use dozens of times every day… and their patients never hear until they're sitting in front of their provider trying to understand what's happening with their body.

This isn't only true in the medical field. Many fields have their own jargon. In my own field, we have phrases such as "cognitive dissonance," "internal family systems" and "acute affective dysregulation." Architects, engineers, hairdressers, pilots, accountants… they all have their own specialized language that doesn't always translate for people who aren't in that field.

Some patients have enough experience with healthcare – either professionally or due to health issues – to pick up on this foreign language. But others are completely naïve to it. And if they struggle with communication or language issues in their native language, understanding this new one is even harder. (And don't even get me started about the challenges patients face for whom English is a second language and medical terminology is now a third language, all happening in the same visit while discussing their health issues; it's a wonder effective care ever happens in those circumstances.)

Several of the patients I interviewed mentioned this challenge with communication. Lona shared her recommendation for how to phrase things more clearly: "'Why am I having my blood drawn?' 'Well, we have these panels to see if you have sugar in your blood or if you have too much fat in your blood.' Simple explanations. 'These things are for this, so we can tell if you need this medication that's going to help with the symptoms you're having.' A little more broken down, you know?"

Clarity

Another factor that the provider brings to the communication equation is clarity… or lack thereof. This factor isn't specific to healthcare communications; clarity is key in effective communication of all kinds. Anyone who's tried to explain the new haircut they want to a barber or hairdresser without a picture to show them knows this. Anyone who's talked to a contractor about what they want done in their kitchen remodel (again, without visual aids) knows this. And any couple who has argued about who was supposed to cook dinner that night knows it, too.

A patient can leave an appointment thinking they know exactly what their new medication regimen is and when and with whom they're supposed to follow up, and their understanding can be completely different than what the care team thought they conveyed. Perhaps more commonly, the patient may be a little confused but because of temperament, the inherent power differential, or cultural issues, they don't ask for clarification. As the quote attributed to Irish playwright George Bernard Shaw points out, "The single biggest problem in communication is the illusion that it has taken place."

Speaking clearly means you've already thought of the likely questions a patient could have and answered or explained them in the most basic, clear, and succinct way possible, before the patient even has the chance to ask. This doesn't mean giving the patient an eight-minute monologue. Using too many words - especially when someone is anxious, surprised, or uncomfortable - is overwhelming and decreases the likelihood that key information will be retained. Use the fewest words to convey the information you need to convey; choose words that are used in everyday language; and repeat the key points.

Clarity also includes instructions for follow-up or next steps. This is a common area where misunderstandings happen, and patients are lost to care. Coral Paris, a retired RN who spent over 50 years working in healthcare, noted, "The visit summaries and handouts are even hard for me sometimes to understand what I'm supposed to do next." As an example, consider this concluding sentence for an outpatient visit:

> *"I'll see you in a few weeks after your lab results come in so we can review them."*

Sounds clear enough, right? Now put yourself in the position of a healthcare-naïve patient and you can see what's missing from the message. Am I supposed to schedule on my way out? Or are they going to call me after my results are in? Do I schedule for a few weeks from today, or a few weeks after the results have already come back?

Now consider this alternative:

> *"Check out at the front desk and schedule a follow-up appointment with me for three weeks from now. Get your lab work done by next week, and at the next appointment we'll go over the results."*

Naturalistic language

This is a good time to talk about naturalistic language. You can think of it as everyday conversational language; this is essentially what I mean when I talk about an absence of jargon. This isn't just helpful in verbal and written communication that's directed to the patient, this can also be helpful for your documentation.

At the time of writing this book, the "open notes" movement has strong momentum, and I suspect will become an accepted best practice in the not-too-distant future. The open notes movement essentially advocates for patients to have immediate open access to their provider's visit documentation. Some of us practice in healthcare systems that support this via patient portals. While this idea still generates a fair bit of anxiety in providers who aren't used to it, it can be a powerful tool. Relevant to this book, open notes are most effective when providers can retrain themselves to document in naturalistic language while still capturing the information they need for the medical record.

Communication: The patient side

Literacy

What do you think the reading comprehension level is of the average adult in the United States? 10th grade? 7th grade?

More than half of Americans (54%) between the ages of 16 and 74 read *below* the 6th grade level. [39,40]

Contrast this with the recommendation from the AMA, the NIH, and the CDC that medical information for the public should be written at no higher than an 8th grade reading level. At an 8th grade level, more than half of our patients will be missing key information because of challenges reading and comprehending our patient materials.

On top of this, about a fifth of Americans – 2 out of 10 – are functionally non-literate or read at a "below-basic" level. At the below-basic level, a person can complete a form with basic information and identify a single piece of information within a short passage.

This is relevant to our discussion of socioeconomic status because literacy levels are correlated with income. [40] The lower the annual income, the lower the average literacy. Of course, this is a bit of a chicken-and-egg topic: Do people have lower literacy levels as a result of their low income? Or do low literacy levels contribute to lower income? Likely both play a role. But it's important to note that the relationship between income and literacy holds true even when other relevant factors are adjusted out, such as age, gender, race/ethnicity, urbanicity, parental education, etc. [40]

Information presented verbally can be just as challenging. Focus and attention decrease when you're anxious; how many of our patients are anxious when we're giving them new information about their health? Lona advised the medical team to put themselves in the patient's shoes, "Being sick is already scary. And going to the doctor is already kind of scary." Once you add in people with auditory processing disorder, low levels of verbal comprehension, or mild hearing loss, a purely auditory presentation isn't going to work for a good chunk of our patients. "Sure," you may be thinking, "I know that, it's why I have handouts." Not only that, but you're a conscientious provider who follows the AMA recommendation not to write medical information for the public any higher than an 8th grade reading level....

Grab your handouts and give them to your 10-year-old niece or nephew, the 2nd grader down the street, or that short person staring at a screen in your own living room. Ask them to read it and then check their comprehension of the material and their understanding of how to apply it in their own life. In a little bit, we'll talk about specific strategies you can incorporate into your practice to accommodate the range of our patients' abilities. I'll also give you some real-life examples of how assumptions about people's abilities are never safe.

Health Literacy

My senior year in college, I got sick. Sicker than I'd ever been. For days, I had a high fever, nausea, struggling to breathe, coughing violently, not able to keep down food or even water. I didn't have insurance and couldn't afford a medical bill, but my roommate and my boyfriend finally convinced me to go to the ER. In the exam room, the young doc went through the usual list of symptoms. When he asked about diarrhea, I said no. He concluded I must be throwing up because my gag reflex was being triggered by the coughing. Then it occurred to me: My bowel movements had been much softer than usual the last couple of days. Did that count as "diarrhea"? My only real reference at that point was the explosive kind that struck at inconvenient moments on sitcoms. The doc started to leave, and in my semi-delirious state I started to panic: Did I give him the wrong information? Is the consistency of my Number 2 critical for his diagnosis? As he headed out the door I blurted, "My poop has been kind of soft - is that diarrhea?" He looked at me sharply: Why is she changing her answer? Why is she pretending she doesn't know what diarrhea is?

When he came back with my chest x-ray, I told him I had thrown up in the garbage can.

"Because you had a coughing fit, right?"

"No, I just felt sick and threw up."

"Because you were coughing."

"No."

He ignored me. I don't know exactly what he thought was happening. Would someone really come to the ER drug-seeking for an anti-emetic?

Health literacy is different than the sort of literacy we discussed above. When the doctor looked at me, he saw a bright, well-educated college student. My ignorance about a basic GI symptom seemed incongruent... and therefore suspicious. This is also a great example of confirmation bias, which we'll be talking about a little later.

On the other hand, visualize a woman who fits your personal stereotype of a multigenerational low SES woman: her personality, her grooming, her communication style. Now imagine that although she quit school after the 9th grade to work a minimum wage job, she has the medical vocabulary and knowledge that would rival any 3rd year med student.

How did this happen? Over the years, she's been the designated caregiver for several family members: Her son with juvenile diabetes and orthopedic problems; her father with chronic cardiac issues; her grandmother with several rounds of cancer and eventually dementia. She's a dedicated caregiver with enough distrust of authority that she always wants to have the information to make her own judgment. Her health literacy vastly exceeds her traditional literacy and formal education.

For a long time, definitions of health literacy focused on an individual's ability to obtain and understand basic health information. In 2020, the US government updated the definition with the Healthy People 2030 initiative. [41] Now the definition includes two distinct parts: Personal health literacy and organizational health literacy.

Personal health literacy is defined as the degree to which an individual has the ability to find, understand, and use information and services to inform health-related decisions and actions for themselves and others. Organizational health literacy is the degree to which organizations equitably enable individuals to find, understand, and use information and services to inform health-related decisions and actions for themselves and others.

The focus isn't just on the person's ability to understand health-related information, such as, "what counts as diarrhea?" It's also their ability to use that information in a way that will benefit them, along with their understanding of medical services and the ability to access them. And it now includes a responsibility on health care organizations to make sure their information and services are accessible and understandable to all people.

My example above includes a bit of both. I certainly came into that situation with a low level of health-related vocabulary; the provider also did a pretty poor job of recognizing my lack of understanding and taking the opportunity to educate me.

Our healthcare system is large and complex. Making it easier to navigate – particularly for those with the lowest level of health literacy – is part of an organization's responsibility. Just call the phone line decision-tree for a large healthcare system and imagine it from the patient's perspective. Am I seeking "primary" or "specialty" care for the issue I'm calling about? Do I need to talk to my doctor, the scheduler, the referral department, or the MA? If I have a question about which medication is covered by my insurance, do I call my provider, the pharmacy, or my insurance company first? Why is there more than one imaging department, and which one do I need? And what the heck is nephrology?

Interestingly, most of the medical providers I interviewed for this book identified health literacy as an area in which their own SES impacted their medical care. (Remember, SES includes occupation.) The clinicians that the providers saw for their own care changed their communication style when they knew they were treating a medical professional. They offered them data and journal articles; they skimmed over basic information they assumed the provider-patients already knew. Which makes sense, right? But they also assumed a high level of health literacy when it didn't exist. Providers described having to ask their clinicians to explain things at a more basic level because it was a specialty area in which they had no experience. One person even said someone in her dental office assumed that because she was a physician she understood dental procedures!

If you're interested in exploring the topic of health literacy further, I'd recommend starting with the CDC's health literacy website. [42] It includes good educational information as well as organizational self-assessments and toolkits.

The Interaction

In the sections above, I made a distinction between care team communication and patient communication. However, these don't live in a vacuum. Communication is an interactive process, with each participant influencing the other in overt and subtle ways on a moment-to-moment basis – sometimes within nanoseconds. A systematic review focused on studies examining communication differences based on patient SES. They found some consistent differences in the communication patterns between providers and high SES patients, and providers and low SES patients. [43]

Results indicated that when interacting with lower SES patients, providers made fewer positive socio-emotional utterances and used a more directive and less participatory communication style. They were less likely to give the patient information and guidance, and made fewer comments designed to build a partnership with the patient. But the difference wasn't only on the provider side. Patients with a lower SES were more passive in their communication and had lower levels of affective expression than higher SES patients did.

It's easy to imagine how these patterns could become a self-perpetuating cycle, starting on either side of the patient-provider equation. For example, a provider is less verbally warm toward their low SES patient; the patient perceives this and reacts by being less emotionally expressive during the visit, which leads the provider to make fewer partnership-building efforts. Or the patient comes into the appointment with a more passive and less communicative style, which leads the provider to perceive them as less invested in their healthcare and to give them less information and guidance.

The power differential

Many conscientious medical personnel pride themselves on being approachable, on connecting with their patients, on showing up in the exam room as a human being rather than the elevated expert showering wisdom down on the ignorant patient. The best ones (in my humble opinion) attempt to generate an egalitarian relationship with the person sitting in front of them. They recognize that while they bring expertise and skill that the patient doesn't have, the patient also brings specialty knowledge they don't have: awareness of their own body, its symptoms, history, reactions, etc. Both sets of knowledge are critical for effective care.

Despite efforts to create a collaborative relationship, there's one factor that is inescapable: the inherent power differential between the provider and patient. It's based on many things, such as the knowledge the provider has that the patient doesn't, the status afforded to medical providers in our society, and the fact that the interaction is taking place on the provider's "turf," a medical setting. For low SES patients, the power differential is all the greater due to the significant difference in social status and value assigned to each in our culture.

For healthcare professionals who pride themselves on their ability to build collaborative relationships with patients, or who come from a disenfranchised background themselves, it can be harder to recognize that the power differential still exists in their practice. PA Spadone put it this way: "I think sometimes as providers, we have all this power. We put that white coat on and we have the stethoscope… Sometimes we forget that in the day-to-day grind."

A power differential can exist the other way, too: When the patient has more social or economic power than the provider or care team does. Imagine your patient has dramatically more wealth, prestige, or social standing than you do. Perhaps they're a celebrity or an artist you're a fan of; perhaps they're a high-ranking political figure; perhaps their name is on the building you're practicing in. Perhaps they're your boss's boss. This power differential can influence your interactions just as much as when it's in the other direction.

The difference in power and status can influence a lower SES patient's willingness to disclose some of the realities of their life. Darlene described it this way: "There's this distance when you perceive that people have more money and resources than you, you have a harder time opening up about where you're at."

It can also impact a patient's ability to advocate for themselves. Imagine you're sitting in a specialist's exam room. It's not a specialty you've had any professional experience with. This is the third time you've come in for the same problem and it's not getting any better. The provider again suggests an intervention you've tried before… But this would be the third time you've been down that same road. The last two times weren't helpful. You're getting frustrated: with the symptoms, their impact on your life, the lack of progress, and not understanding what could be gained by trying the exact same thing again. And the intervention is not easy. It'll take time, effort, money, and potential side effects. Do you go along with what they recommended? Do you give up altogether and just deal with the symptoms? Or do you express your concern and ask for a different approach?

Now, recall the earlier discussion regarding common narratives we apply to lower SES patients: They don't come in and they don't care. Is it possible that the patient you're applying these narratives to simply has a disagreement, or concern, or need that they don't feel comfortable bringing up directly? The patients I interviewed recalled times when they simply didn't follow up with a provider or a recommendation if they felt it wasn't a good fit for them, rather than talk about it directly. As Darlene put it, "I know for me, I've sat there and I was like, 'Okay, yep,' and in my mind I already knew."

Perhaps it's the power differential that underlies the difference in communication between providers and lower SES patients versus higher SES patients. This difference in power can be subtle and sneaky and contribute to a cycle that reinforces stereotypes. When the interaction seems "off," or when you find yourself applying negative stereotypes or narratives, or when treatment simply isn't progressing the way you expect, Dr. Whittier recommends, "Taking that moment to pause, sort of like an eye-opener that there's something else going on, it's not just about me writing a prescription, it's not just about me saying 'I need you to.'"

One antidote to the potential negative impact that can result from the power differential is called "power sharing." It's just what it sounds. Clinical decisions are shared between the care team and the patient. Interventions are chosen based on both the best evidence and the values and preferences of the patient. Treatment plans are purposefully tailored to the patients' individual needs. This isn't simple; in some ways it contradicts the traditional "expert" role of the care team as well as the implicit training patients receive not to question the authority of the doctor or the nurse.

Power sharing in medicine can also refer to sharing power within and across the care team. This includes giving nurses, MAs, clerks, trainees, and all members the power to make observations, bring up concerns, and contribute information. In the larger sense, power sharing is about valuing the contribution of everyone involved: The provider, every member of the care team, the patient, and the patients' advocates. It's simple in theory, but in practice is harder to implement and ensure it's being experienced the way it's intended. Dr. Cucalon Calderon advocates a first step: "Just being open to learn from the people in front of you as to how they do things and recognizing that they are going to be the leaders in their own experience."

In this chapter, we've covered a lot of information about the complex "why" that might explain the difference between caring providers' interactions, assessments, and treatment decisions with high SES versus low SES patients. This time, the reflection questions are divided between the different topics we discussed.

Reflection

Narratives:

1) Think about your earliest training experiences: What explanations, attributions or stories were told about lower SES patients?

2) Which narratives do you recognize as ones you've told yourself or passed on to others?

Population data versus individual data:

3) Can you remember an experience with a patient when you were surprised by a discrepancy between what you expected to find (based on SES-related population data) and the patient's actual history or presentation?

Communication:

4) Observe your language during your next few conversations with patients. Try to identify words or phrases you use on a regular basis that make perfect sense to you and your co-workers but might not to a healthcare-naïve patient. What "everyday" words could you use instead?

Power differential:

5) When do you find it easy to share power with patients? When is it harder? Certain patients, certain problems, certain settings, certain risks?

PART 3:
What Can You Do About It?
Reducing the Impact on Patient Care

CHAPTER 8
Common (not-so-helpful) Responses

Sometimes they look at people that are like, homeless or on Medicaid and they don't have a job or what have you, they treat you a little bit different. They judge you, they think you're a drug addict, they aren't – a lot of them aren't very kind.

- LONA S.

Before we jump into specific strategies, let's talk about some reactions I've observed across a range of healthcare professionals when working with disenfranchised patients. Let me be clear: I don't present these to judge or wag my finger. These are common, very human reactions. Some are based on the hard-wiring of our cognitive systems, some on our own life experiences, and some on our professional experience. Below are several of the most common ones I've seen. As you read, pay attention to which ones resonate with your experience.

Avoid it altogether

The most basic response is to simply avoid the topic of a patient's socioeconomic challenges. You're not a social worker, right? You can fulfill your role without knowing the patient's employment status, housing situation, or how high their credit card debt is.

Medical professionals avoid this topic in a variety of ways and for a variety of reasons: It's uncomfortable, it doesn't feel like their place, they don't have the knowledge, time, or resources to address it. Dr. Larson empathized, "I understand why my colleagues don't want to do it [ask about patients' living circumstances]. Because they want to solve problems and if they can't, they just feel bad."

A few of the patients I interviewed indicated that when a medical office or healthcare system doesn't ask any questions related to their socioeconomics, they assume the topic is off limits because the provider doesn't understand the impact, doesn't think it's relevant, or perhaps doesn't care. But one patient had a different take on it. When I asked Chad if he had experienced times when medical professionals didn't "get it" about his socioeconomic challenges, he had this response: "I think they do get it, but they're at a loss of what to do. So, it may come across as 'don't get it' but they're out of options. What do you do when you truly believe there's nothing you can do?"

Experiential gap

It can be hard putting yourself in someone else's shoes if you haven't shared similar experiences. It's part of human nature to see the world through our own lenses without even being aware that we're wearing them. I'm calling this difference the "experiential gap": the gap that may exist between your socioeconomic experiences and those of your lower SES patients, and the lack of awareness that often results.

There are some key areas I've observed where this experiential gap is likely to show up, and some key experiences that are common for low SES folks but hard to grasp if you haven't experienced it yourself. On the provider's side, one of the clues that we're dealing with an experiential gap is when reasons are dismissed as excuses.

Take, for example, the patient who insists that they "can't take time off work" to attend an appointment. The sad fact is many people do not have access to sick time or paid leave for medical care. So whatever time is spent somewhere other than work is a direct loss of wages. And if you have a co-pay or deductible for the appointment, not only are you not getting paid but you're spending money. "But the appointment isn't long," you think, "It's only a couple of hours. It's not like you have to take a whole day off." However, if you do shift work, you may in fact have to take a whole day off so that your position is covered. If you work on a production line in a small business, as a server in a busy restaurant, or as the only clerk in a small retail store, your time away from your task must be covered. And that often means coverage for your entire shift; otherwise, you're asking another employee to interrupt their day off to come into work for just a couple of hours. (And let's face it; medical appointments don't always run perfectly on time, so will you actually be back to work in two hours? Two and a half? Three?) In many cases, if the employee has to miss a scheduled shift, they're also responsible for finding their own coverage. So, to attend that simple appointment, you have to first find someone to take your shift for you, and then lose an entire day of pay.

Another area where an experiential gap shows up is around available time. We often hear patients say they don't have time to exercise, take care of preventative care, monitor their glucose or blood pressure, etc. "How can you not have time to go for a simple 10-minute walk? It's not like I'm asking you to exercise for an hour a day." But if you're getting the kids up and ready for school early in the morning, dropping them at the before-school program, heading to Job #1 from 8:00am-5:00pm, picking up the kids, making dinner, helping with homework, getting them settled with the neighbor who watches them at night, and then heading to job #2 from 9:00pm-1:00am… Squeezing in a ten minute walk is nearly impossible. It's a similar situation for a patient who has responsibility for managing the appointments and needs of both children and other family members. If you have high demands and limited time, the choice becomes what you sacrifice: Your parent's appointment with their oncologist, or your appointment for that nagging stomach issue you've been dealing with?

Similarly, the environmental barriers discussed earlier – a safe environment, reliable and accessible transportation, access to healthy and affordable food – are all realities that are easy to dismiss as excuses. That's certainly not to say that the patient's medical needs aren't critically important. It's about whether an "excuse" reflects the reality of their situation.

Let me just take a moment to acknowledge how hard it is to hear these reasons over and over, even if you recognize how real they are. If you work with economically disadvantaged patients, some days it feels like every conversation you have is about why someone didn't get their lab work done, or keeps showing up in your ER for the same problem, or never followed up on the referral… And meanwhile, you can clearly see the future consequences of the choices the patient is making now.

As noted above, PA Spadone has spent her entire career working with disenfranchised patients. Even with those years of experience, she described a recent experience with a patient that reminded her not to make assumptions:

> Last month I had a patient I had known for many years… I added a blood pressure medicine for him. I said, 'Okay, go downstairs [to the pharmacy] and get your blood pressure medicine and come back in two weeks.' So, he comes back in two weeks and there's no change in his blood pressure. So I ask him, 'How come there's no change? Are you taking the medicine?' And he tells me, 'Oh no, two weeks ago I didn't have the money to get it. Tomorrow I get paid, tomorrow I'll get it.' But that wasn't a conversation that happened before. In my mind, I was like, 'Simple. High blood pressure medicine that's only four bucks.' For you and I, it's not a problem, but for him, he couldn't afford the four dollars.

The experience reminded her to add financial information to her patient education. She gave the example, "This is a high blood pressure medicine, it's generic, you should be able to get it for four dollars, if you cannot afford it right now let me know…"

It's hard to hold both truths at the same time: The patient's barriers are real and often insurmountable, and the medical consequences - if they could just find a way around those barriers - are completely preventable.

This experiential gap also extends to the other end of the socioeconomic continuum. For our most affluent patients, it can be just as hard for us to envision – or take seriously – the challenges and barriers they face. It's easy to give in to the thought, "If I had that much money…" But imagine you're the head of a Fortune 500 company that hasn't been performing well. Now you must report on the third consecutive bad quarter. The last thing you need is for your board of directors to discover you've been attending more medical appointments than usual and get suspicious that you have a developing health issue you're going to be "distracted" by. You may show up at the next board meeting to a vote of no confidence and be out of a job. Postponing medical care may feel like the only option to protect your career.

Narrative contagion

Another common reaction is to reinforce the narratives that have been passed down to us, as described earlier. This can happen the way narratives are often passed down: Through stories told, attributions made, and off-hand comments. But there's another way narratives can be passed along that's even more powerful: through our documentation. Embedding these narratives about low SES patients in how we document is especially dangerous for two reasons. One, because it follows the patient and influences the perception of anyone reading that note. Two, because we give more weight to things when they're in writing.

How do these negative narratives get included in documentation? Sometimes it's subtle and sometimes not. Early in my training working on an inpatient psychiatric unit, there was a patient with an extensive trauma history who was having frequent dissociative episodes. They were clearly overwhelming for her and very disruptive to the functioning of the unit. One of the psychiatrists, frustrated with the situation and feeling powerless to fix it, wrote in her chart, "Patient is HOLDING THE ENTIRE UNIT HOSTAGE with her acting-out behavior and histrionics." Yikes. Not too subtle, and that entry lived in that patient's chart for every future provider to see.

More subtle versions often involve our choice of words. Did the patient "refuse" or did they "decline"? Are they "non-compliant," or "non-adherent," or did they "opt not to at this time"? Did they "again neglect to follow-up"? Sometimes our phrasing can include a scolding or condescending or frustrated tone, or imply that we don't believe the reasons the patient gave us or don't take them seriously.

PA Spadone recommends a matter-of-fact documentation style that includes the key information without any damaging narrative undertones. She gives the example: "Patient really needs an ultrasound. However, patient has informed me that he is not able to afford $700 for the ultrasound. The risks of not getting an ultrasound were discussed with the patient." And then, she says, you should help find resources for the patient to get the ultrasound.

Minimize differences

SES – at least the income part – can be relative within any given professional group, and that's true for medical providers. Advanced practice clinicians (APRNs and PAs) have a far lower income than MDs or DOs. And a physician working in academia or a community health center makes far less money than their colleague in a lucrative private practice. Medical students and residents often feel "poor," and relative to what their income will be when they're practicing, they are.

It's hard-wired into the human brain to make comparisons and put people into different boxes and categories. One way of addressing our own discomfort in recognizing the challenges our low SES patients face is to minimize the differences between us and them. Jokes about being broke because we work in academia, or calling yourself a poor resident, talking about the level of debt you have because of student loans or how old your car is or how small your house is – these all may have some truth to them. But at their core, they're often an attempt to avoid the distress of truly recognizing the reality of our patients' lives.

Feeling badly... and the sequalae

You've been working with patient James for many years, and you know him pretty well. He comes to a follow-up visit and tells you he's lost his job and is about to get evicted from his apartment. He's not sure how he's going to pay for his medications. You like James; he's a pleasant guy, a hard worker, and very earnest in his efforts to improve his health. You direct him to the discount program that's available for some of his medications, ask if he's applying for unemployment and other benefits. He seems to be doing everything he can to solve his situation.

By his next visit things have gotten worse. He lost his apartment and is now sleeping on the couch at his nephew's. It's a fifth-floor walk-up; the nephew and his roommates all drink a lot and use various substances. James isn't sleeping and he's only filling his most critical prescriptions. He's applying for jobs, but at his age hasn't gotten any good leads.

Most people would feel bad for James in this situation. And – depending on your own personality and inclinations – this feeling might lead you in a few different directions.

Over-helping

Many people who go into healthcare have a heart for helping, and seeing people suffer without doing something about it goes against their nature. This instinct to help is like many things in life: There's an optimal amount that is healthy for both the helper and the recipient. Too little helpful drive isn't great, and too much can lead to problems. For this section, we're talking about the "too much" side of the continuum. If this isn't you, you've probably known someone who takes their helping instinct into what we behavioral health folks refer to as "boundary issues."

The challenge is that it can start small and just look like admirable altruism. In fact, we often reward this type of behavior. Think of the provider who takes time at the end of the day to contact their pharmaceutical rep and see if there are other options for James' meds. Or the MA who texts their social worker friend to ask about housing options they can refer James to. We admire their compassion and often recognize these folks for going above and beyond. Don't get me wrong, there's nothing wrong with that. These are not the people I'm talking to now.

Suppose the pharmaceutical rep can't help, and none of the housing options work out, and James is still living with his verbally abusive nephew who is now having drunken fights with his girlfriend at three o clock every morning. His blood pressure is up, his glucose is getting out of control, and his latest depression screen is worrying. Imagine you're now talking to James on the phone every week. You've suggested he see a counselor, but of course he can't afford one. So, you decide to loan him a little money to get out of his situation. And you're concerned about his mental health, so you start texting him every day just to check in. One small loan leads to the next, but you know he'll pay you back, and you tell yourself that as soon as he has a therapist you can stop worrying about him so much. James is so grateful. He seems a little embarrassed when he comes in for his visits now, but it feels good to be helping someone out in the real world of their life where you can't usually make a difference. That powerless feeling is finally gone.

Some of the providers I interviewed talked about the temptation – and the risks – of helping patients who are trying hard but still facing significant barriers. Dr. Larson said, "I never did open my pocketbook at work. I thought about it a whole bunch, but I thought, 'You know, if you open that door, that's not going to work.' I donate in other ways."

More generally, Dr. Whittier talked about both the benefits and risks of developing a close relationship with our patients. Building a sense of trust helps patients feel comfortable disclosing important information. But it also means they may begin to perceive the relationship as a friendship that can cross professional boundaries. "That's not helpful to them or me," Dr. Whittier observed. "Figuring out what you can help, what you can't help, and how to keep those boundaries all at the same time. It can be very tricky."

Guilt

Awareness of the dramatic difference between our life circumstance and some of our patients' can lead to a sense of guilt. This can be exacerbated if we feel we're not grateful enough for what we have, or if we've made judgmental assumptions about our patients, or recognize that our behaviors with our lower SES patients haven't been the best. It can also take the form of "survivor guilt" if you come from a similar background as your patients, or if your SES is significantly higher than your family of origin or community of origin.

There was a saying that was popular some years ago: "Guilt is a useless emotion." I understand the helpful intention behind this but as a psychologist, I can't endorse it. I believe that feeling guilty over things that you had no part in and have no control over is useless. If you feel personally guilty about a typhoon that happened half a world away, or the fact that your cousin has cancer, or that you don't have the ability to solve all your patients' socioeconomic problems… that's pretty useless. But I think there's such a thing as realistic guilt. And I think it can be pretty darn helpful if you pay attention to it.

Sometimes feeling guilty – realistic guilt – is a sign that we've violated our own ethics and beliefs, or those that we genuinely value from our family or our culture. This feeling of guilt is a signal. It's telling us that we should pay attention to our actions and address them in some way: learn from the situation, make amends, or fix whatever is triggering the guilt. If we realize that our past behavior with low SES patients was less than ideal, this might be realistic guilt. It's our own brain's way of telling us it's time to make a change.

Powerlessness

In the face of our patients' suffering – or the world's suffering, for that matter – it's hard not to feel a sense of powerlessness. The problems are big, there are rarely easy solutions, and our own ability to effect change is limited. This experience of powerlessness can lead to burnout, compassion fatigue, learned helplessness and moral distress.

There's been a lot written about burnout and compassion fatigue. More recently, the topic of moral distress has been getting attention, particularly in the nursing field. Moral distress in healthcare is when there's a conflict between what we believe is the ethical thing to do and what we're required to do based on our role, regulations, or policy. An example may be your belief that patients who can't afford their medication should be given samples, but your clinic leadership has enacted a policy against using them. Or if clinical guidelines and your professional experience tell you a patient needs a specific treatment, but their insurance company refuses to cover it and your institution won't write it off.

You may be less familiar with the concept of learned helplessness; this is a well-researched phenomenon from the field of psychology. Explained simply, learned helplessness is what results when efforts to escape from a negative stimulus repeatedly fail. When a person learns – over many attempts – that their efforts make no difference and they have zero control, they experience a state of helplessness. Here's the interesting part, though: If you then present them with an obvious means to escape or to change the situation, they don't take it. It's as if they no longer have the ability to recognize that escape is possible. That's learned helplessness.

I imagine this as the state some healthcare professionals find themselves in. The unpleasant stimulus is the sadness, frustration, or powerlessness they feel about a patient's situation. So they attempt to find a resource to help the patient, or they try to set up appropriate follow-up before the patient is discharged from the hospital, or they only prescribe generics so their patients can fill their prescriptions… And it doesn't work. Over and over, despite their best efforts, it doesn't change the outcome. Then when a new opportunity presents itself that might yield a different outcome: a new referral resource, a highly motivated patient, expanded payer benefits… it isn't even seen.

Defensiveness and Blame

Humans are built to defend ourselves against threats, both physical and psychological. If a ball is coming toward our face, our hands reflexively come up and we move our head out of the way before we even consciously register the impending blow. The same thing happens with emotional and psychological threats. Someone hurls an unexpected insult, and we reflexively defend ourselves: By refuting it, by insulting them back, by dismissing it before we even assess whether it's true.

Recognizing the vast SES-related inequities in the world can feel threatening, whether we explicitly recognize this or not. It can threaten our view of the world, our belief system, our own sense of security for ourselves or the people we love. There are many ways we can defend ourselves from this threat: We can refuse to see the inequities or minimize them. We can defend the system that's being blamed for creating them. We also can blame the person who is in that situation.

A common way to defend ourselves is to find reasons why it makes sense that this person is in dire financial straits. Humans are wired to find explanations. Present someone with an ambiguous situation, and they will generate a story to explain it and make it make sense. Even for our own life histories, we generate stories to explain why we are the way we are: I'm an only child; I had a particular formative experience in my youth; my parents did (or did not) do x, y, and z; my ex treated me such-and-such a way; I'm a Gemini. That's not to say that the reasons aren't valid and accurate. It's just helpful to recognize that our brains are more comfortable when 1) we have a reason for why things happen, and 2) that reason fits into our worldview.

When we're presented with a situation that challenges us – people suffer and lack adequate resources – our brains do their job and find an explanation for why that is. And so long as our brain is generating a reason, why not generate one that holds the person responsible for their situation, which reassures us that we're protected from the same fate?

It's often this reason-finding that leads us to "blame the victim" for their circumstances. If they're in this situation because they made poor choices, weren't motivated, didn't work hard, didn't take advantage of opportunities we certainly would have taken advantage of… Then we have a nice clean explanation for why the world is the way it is. And why we won't find ourselves in the same dire circumstance.

This tendency to blame the victim is exacerbated if the person we're finding an explanation about belongs to a group that already has negative stereotypes associated with them. In that case, our brain doesn't even need to work to find an explanation; it's already there, just waiting for an opportunity to pop up and provide the explanation. In my experience, it often goes like this: [insert specific individual] is in this situation because [insert specific group] are [insert negative characteristic]. This can be one of those implicit biases that exist outside of conscious awareness. "That woman is sleeping in her car because homeless people are all drug addicts." *Stereotype + need for the world to make sense = blame.*

This is a good point to talk about one of my favorite concepts from the field of social psychology. I genuinely believe that if everyone learned this research, internalized it, and got good at recognizing it, the world would be a better place.

The self-serving bias in attribution

Attribution is about how we explain why people do what they do. For example, if we're driving down the freeway and we see someone in our rearview mirror speeding and weaving through traffic, then zooming up and cutting in front of us to go across two lanes to take an exit, to what do we attribute this behavior? In other words, what are we thinking about that driver (or muttering, or hollering out the window)? We might think they're a terrible driver, or a jerk, or a selfish person who thinks that getting where they're going is more important than other people's safety.

But what if we're the person driving fast, changing lanes to pass everyone we can, and cutting across traffic to make our exit? We aren't likely thinking of ourselves as a terrible driver who doesn't care about other people's safety, right? When we do it, it's because we're running late for an urgent appointment, the lights were all red, and we're just trying to get around those stupid slow drivers who are holding everybody up.

In other words, we're more likely to attribute other people's bad behavior to an internal cause – their personality, lack of self-control, irresponsibility, or just plain stupidity, for example. At the same time, we're more likely to attribute our own bad behavior to an external cause – bad luck, circumstances outside our control, or other people's influence. Conversely, we tend to attribute our own successes to internal factors (hard work, talent), and other's successes to external factors (luck, the help of others).

This is called the Self-Serving Bias in Attribution, or "self-serving bias" for short. It's a robust finding in social psychology. [44]

Think of any recent situation. When we see a parent raising their voice at their kid in the grocery store, it's because they don't know how to control their anger. When we raise our voice at our kid in the grocery store, it's because we had the worst day and our kid is pushing our buttons on purpose. If our co-worker is late to an important meeting, it's because they aren't reliable; if we're late to an important meeting, it's because the previous meeting ran long. Applied to low-socioeconomic status patients, we may be making assumptions about the causes of their behavior that we wouldn't make if it were our own same behavior.

What if I recognized myself in this chapter?

As I said in the introduction to this chapter, all these reactions, though less-than-helpful, are also quite common. The key is in recognizing them and then working to eliminate them, or at least minimize their impact on our clinical work and our interactions with patients.

That said, some folks will find it harder to move beyond their implicit or explicit biases when working with patients living in a lower socioeconomic position. If you have a negative visceral reaction to specific patients, if you cannot find empathy, if you've diligently read this book and done the exercises and still find yourself unable to move beyond your biases… You're human. But don't let yourself off the hook; keep at it. And in the meantime, ensure those patients are getting good care by referring them to a trusted colleague.

Reflection

1) Of the responses and reactions described in this chapter – avoidance, lack of understanding, minimizing differences, over-helping, guilt, powerlessness, blame, and the self-serving bias – which ones did you recognize in yourself, either currently or in the past?

2) Which of these reactions have you seen or heard from co-workers and colleagues?

3) Part of addressing these reactions is figuring out where we have control and where we don't. When it comes to the struggles of our patients, how can you have a positive influence that's still within the bounds of your professional role?

CHAPTER 9
Change Is Hard... And Possible

It's not anything I had experienced, so I had to learn.

– Dr. Trudy Larson

One of my pet peeves is when a speaker or author spends hours or pages talking about a problem... and then doesn't offer any specific recommendations or solutions. I'm not saying there isn't value in deep dives into theoretical topics, or research that identifies a previously unrecognized problem, or a summary of the current state of knowledge in some area. But if there are solutions to be had, let's have them.

A clinical supervisor of mine once told me, "Insight is a booby prize." This may sound surprising coming from a psychologist – it was to me at the time. But he meant that insight without change isn't worth much. So far, we've covered what SES is, the impact on patients' healthcare experience, possible reasons for that impact, and common provider reactions. Embedded throughout these chapters have been ideas, suggestions, and insights to help you begin modifying your mind and your practice. The final part of this book is even more focused on explicit recommendations. I've divided the strategies into what I'm calling "external" and "internal" strategies.

The external strategies are practical in nature. These interventions and suggestions focus on the physical environment we're practicing in, the materials that are part of our practice, and how information is communicated. The internal strategies are largely cognitive; they're focused on the perceptions, assumptions, and thought processes that impact our interactions with patients. Of course, there's an overlap between external and internal strategies. In some cases, I've made an arbitrary distinction because the strategy involves both internal and external change.

Before we get into them, a small caveat: Not all strategies will apply equally to all settings, all specialties, or all roles on the care team. Likewise, they won't necessarily apply to all patients. As noted before, patients who might be classified in a lower socioeconomic position are a heterogeneous group. The risk in any list of strategies is implying that everyone in that group is the same and not recognizing the importance of individual differences.

For both the external and internal strategies that follow, I'd ask you to read them with a discerning eye: Which ones will be most applicable for your patients, your practice, and you as a person and a professional? I'm a pragmatist at heart. Use the ones that make sense for you and feel free to ignore the rest.

Reflection

1) On a scale of 1-10, how ready do you feel to make changes in your understanding and approach to lower socioeconomic status patients?

2) What might get in the way of you making those changes?

CHAPTER 10
External Strategies

I know so many people who are just fed up with the way the system works for the individual that they just won't go to a doctor.

- FEATHER C.

I started this project determined to write a book that was concise, easily digestible, and with practical strategies that might require a little effort but were all basically doable. Doable without spending a lot of money, completely overhauling your practice, or adding way more "tools" into your busy day. Hopefully, the strategies in this section meet that goal.

Talking about SES

Toward the end of my pre-doctoral psychology internship year, as part of the formal feedback at the end of a rotation, the supervisor suggested that I should dress "nicer" for work. To be clear, I wasn't wearing ripped jeans and tee shirts. My clothes were well within the "business casual" range. In fairness, they probably weren't the newest looking. My supervisor wasn't trying to be offensive; he was a kind person who believed in the professionalism of the field.

I hid in the bathroom and cried.

What that supervisor didn't know was that I was selling my plasma twice a week to cover my rent. I was getting donated food from food banks. I was going through bankruptcy proceedings.

I had arrived at that financial crisis due to a conflux of circumstances: My internship paid an annual salary that was barely double the federal poverty level, yet they had a strict "no moonlighting" rule. Interns also weren't eligible for health insurance. This was before the Affordable Care Act or the marketplace, so if your job didn't offer insurance, you were out of luck. My husband had recently had emergency surgery; he hadn't been able to work and required frequent ongoing follow-up care. Between unpaid medical bills, overwhelming student loans, and our tiny income, we were drowning.

I certainly didn't have money to go buy a new wardrobe.

The reason my supervisor – and in fact no one at my internship – knew about my financial desperation was simple: I hadn't told them. My workplace was full of kind, supportive people who wanted the best for their bright young intern. If I had told them, I have no doubt they would have found a way to help.

I was too ashamed.

Financial status as a measure of success and competence is strongly woven into our cultural values. Pair that with our value of independence and a "pull yourself up by your bootstraps" expectation, and it becomes hard to admit that you're struggling financially. Even the language we use reflects it – did you hear it in that last sentence? We "admit" that we're financially insecure, as we would admit a wrongdoing. It took many, many years for me to realize that the system had been broken for me, as it is for many people, and that my financial crisis wasn't a personal failure.

It's not safe to assume any aspect of someone's socioeconomic position – income, occupation, or education – unless you have factual knowledge of it. Dr. Larson described the results of a survey at the university where she was teaching: "That was a pretty big deal." The faculty wanted to get a better picture of who the medical students were, their backgrounds, and their life circumstances, so they asked students to complete an anonymous questionnaire. They were shocked to discover the number of students living in poverty; their tuition and books were covered by grants, but they didn't have enough money for food. Many of them were working jobs that interfered with their class schedule so they could pay for their housing.

If you don't ask, you won't find out. Even if you do ask, you may not find out. Aside from embarrassment, our patients may fear potential consequences. If a parent discloses that they and their children are couch-surfing because they lost their housing, they may wonder: Will you report them to child protective services? If a patient discloses that they're working a side job off-the-books to pay for their medication, they may worry they could lose their food stamp benefits.

As hard as these conversations can be, clearly, they're important. There are some specific strategies I'd recommend to increase the odds that a patient will share their economic barriers with you:

1) Introduce the topic with some context: "We ask about many things that can impact your medical care, such as your health conditions, your family background, and your financial and housing situation."

2) Ask in a matter-of-fact way, just as you would ask about any other factor related to a medical condition. For example, "This medicine needs to be taken with food. Do you have enough food at home right now to be able to do that?"

3) If possible, use a questionnaire rather than asking face-to-face; patients may feel more comfortable disclosing in that format.

There are several questionnaires that are designed for medical settings and assess patients' social determinants of health. I've included information about three of them in Appendix A. Of course, once you ask the questions you must be prepared to do something with that information. Not having resources to address the need doesn't help the patient and can add to the care team's sense of helplessness and burnout. In Appendix B, I've included resources, information, and links that can be provided to patients. In a section below, we'll also talk about the care team and how different roles can support this practice.

Standardized language

My younger brother has always been a voracious reader. In his early 20s he read nearly every book in the library. He eagerly devoured *War and Peace*, the 1200+ page classic by Leo Tolstoy. He's a smart guy.

He's also missing several teeth. He hasn't held a formal job in 20 years. The library he read his way through was a prison library. For over a decade, he's lived in a converted school bus in the desert. He's lean, scruffy, and on any given day may not smell the greatest. He still reads everything he can get his hands on, but if he presented in your exam room you'd instinctively "dumb-down" your communication.

Compare this to the successful software engineer with dyslexia and an auditory processing disorder. They're an educated professional with a high SES, but they read at a 7th grade level and will only comprehend about half the information you present to them verbally.

As we've discussed, part of the typical way of defining SES is education level. Given that, our tendency to assume intellectual ability, knowledge, and verbal skills based on a person's SES is understandable. But the risk is in those situations – like the examples above – where there's an incongruence. This happens more often than most people are aware.

Standardizing our language is one way to avoid these sorts of misses. If we generate a clear, simple explanation using naturalistic language for the conversations we have most frequently with patients – not so simple that patients feel condescended to, but simple enough that the majority of people can follow – we can apply these consistently. We'll be less likely to fall prey to assumptions.

Patient education materials and modalities

I love it when I see patients walking out of medical offices and hospitals with handouts. Not everyone learns best via auditory channels, and in the heat of the situation it can be hard to absorb and retain everything. Having information conveyed in more than one modality is a great practice.

Review your handouts for length, format, clarity, and reading level. Based on the recommendations of the AMA, CDC, and NIH, a lot of patient materials are written around the 8th grade reading level. But as we discussed earlier, if we aim for the 5th or 4th grade, or even 3rd, we'll be doing a great service for many of our patients. If the materials include images or pictographs that convey the key points of the text, that's even better.

Giving the patient a link to a website that conveys the information is also a great approach. Let's face it – many of them have already looked up their symptoms or conditions before they see us. We can play a key role in guiding them to a reputable website with trustworthy information. Just be sure you're vetting your favorite websites for clarity and lack of medical jargon. Patient-oriented online videos are an excellent option as well, since they avoid the challenges that can come with text-based information.

Offering information in multiple formats to all our patients minimizes the risk that an assumption or bias is influencing the choice of materials we give to different patients. Simply tell them that you would like to give them more information about the condition/diagnosis/recommendation/treatment options, and ask whether they'd prefer handouts, a link to a website, or an online video. The patient can choose the source that fits best for them without having to acknowledge any weaknesses or deficits.

Checking in

Checking in with a patient for their understanding is critical. Fortunately, most providers have now been trained to do this. The end of most primary care or specialty visits is "Do you have any questions?" While this is a great change from the days of yesteryear when providers just sent patients out the door with the assumption that they understood and would comply, I'd suggest a few modifications to increase the effectiveness.

The first one is a simple change of language. Tweaking a couple of words in our standard phrasing can make a huge difference in whether patients – especially those least likely to advocate for themselves – share what's on their mind. Instead of asking, "Do you have any questions," more effective phrasing is, "What questions do you have for me?" This assumes that there will naturally be questions and that we're expecting to spend time addressing them. It normalizes a conversation about information shared and recommendations given. This must be paired with a relaxed posture and an attentive expression.

This combination of open phrasing plus non-verbal communication invites the patient to consider the information that was discussed and what questions they may have, rather than answering with a reflexive "no." Asking what questions a patient has while looking at a monitor or standing up to leave will not have the desired effect. (Unless the desired effect is to shut down the conversation. Which, with some more loquacious patients, it may be. But use this strategically and judiciously.)

If you want to take it to the next level, then I'd suggest adding one more word: "concerns." As in, "What questions or concerns do you have about what we've talked about?" A patient may not have any questions because they've already decided they don't feel comfortable following your recommendation, can't afford the co-pay, or heard something negative on social media about what you just prescribed. The word "concerns" allows the opportunity to open the conversation about any and all barriers.

Checking in this way seems like it could add time to the visit. And that is a risk; I'm not going to pretend it's not. But it's also a time-saver in many cases. Finding out the questions or concerns during this contact with the patient can prevent: Having to repeat the same conversation at the next appointment, inpatient admission, or ER visit; phone calls to the office staff or MA; messages on the patient portal; or the time it takes to address the worsening issue because the treatment plan wasn't followed to begin with. If time is truly a concern, or you know this is a patient who would love to spend all day talking to you, simple expectation-setting of, "We have a few minutes left, what questions or concerns do you have for me?" can be effective.

Checking in as a regular conclusion to visits is important, but there's one other situation in which it's critical: When the patient is struggling to adhere to the treatment plan. If you notice that you're making the same recommendation repeatedly or things just aren't moving forward in the way you expect, plan to spend a part of your next visit checking in about why. It's easy to fall into the rut of simply repeating your recommendations at each visit – often with a slightly scolding tone. Instead, with a collaborative tone, invite the patient into a discussion, "I'm wondering what's getting in the way of us moving forward on X problem."

As part of the discussion, acknowledge that follow-through is often harder than we think it's going to be. Suggest that if this isn't the right plan, you'd like to work with them to come up with something more realistic. Mention common barriers for other patients: Transportation, time, cost, understanding how the plan will fix the problem, or whether it will be effective. This approach can feel like it's outside of your scope. You're not a therapist or a social worker. But if the goal is to improve patients' health, then you want to use all the tools at your disposal, which includes both the medical tools and the interpersonal ones.

It's also worth mentioning that despite all the medical evidence, health issues, or risks, a patient simply may not want to do the thing that you know will be most helpful. Don't forget to ask the patient if they actually want to address the issue at this time. If not, talk with them about how they'll know when the time is right. As PA Spadone put it, "You want so much for your patients, but they're not ready… You can't force people to do things, just like I don't want people forcing me to do things, right?... We don't know why they're making the choice they're making."

Motivational Interviewing

Speaking of tools, there's a ridiculously effective one that few healthcare professionals are trained in. It's an evidence-based, highly researched approach that helps patients change their health behaviors. Thirty years of studies and meta-analyses have demonstrated that use of this approach – as compared to standard treatment – yields statistically significant improvements in patients' physical activity, alcohol and tobacco use, dental hygiene, body weight, HIV viral load, treatment adherence, willingness to change behavior, and mortality. What is this amazing tool that everyone could use but few do? It's a deceptively simple communication approach called Motivational Interviewing (MI).

MI was developed by clinical psychologists William R. Miller and Stephen Rollnick. The core goals in MI are to assist the patient in connecting with their own intrinsic motivation and capacity for behavior change, resolve their ambivalence, and move from motivation to action. This happens via four core processes: Engaging, Focusing, Evoking, and Planning.

MI works in concert with another useful model, the Transtheoretical Model, also known colloquially as the Stages of Change model. The Transtheoretical Model was developed by James O. Prochaska and Carlo Di Clemente and identifies five stages the patient may be in related to their readiness to make a specific behavior change: Precontemplation, Contemplation, Determination, Action, and Maintenance. An MI approach assists the patient in moving through these stages to develop a sustainable change in a specific health behavior.

If you really want to increase your effectiveness with patients – all patients – I'd recommend finding workshops, workbooks, or continuing education focused on MI for healthcare professionals. The core skills involved seem simple but require training and practice to modify our communication habits. In Appendix C, I've included some websites and links to MI resources.

Care coordination, resource linking, and the care team

In my view, coordination of care is one of the most powerful life-saving activities healthcare personnel can engage in. Effective care coordination can prevent medication interactions, missed diagnoses, under- and over-treatment, contradictory treatment plans, and patients dropping out of care because they're confused or overwhelmed.

Linking patients to resources is equally powerful. Connecting people to social services and community resources that can address social determinants of health makes it possible for you and your patient to attend to their medical needs.

If you work in a medical setting with truly integrated care, then you're ahead of the game. Some community health centers and public health agencies have a care team approach that may include social workers, mental health professionals, and other ancillary services. The providers I interviewed who've worked in these settings were clear about the benefits. "I look at my colleagues and say, 'I don't know how you can do this. If you're in a solo practice, I don't know how you do this,'" said Dr. Larson. PA Spadone echoed this sentiment about providers who work in settings without case management or wrap-around services: "I don't know how they do it. It's super hard."

Providers also highlighted the critical role that each member of the care team plays. Dr. Shane talked about his experience working with an integrated team: "I'll find one thing out, the MA will find something out, then behavioral health will go in and they'll get something completely different. And unless you can all communicate together you never get the full picture." Dr. Larson mentioned this as well, observing, "You never know who on the medical team someone is going to confide in."

Patients also talked about the critical role of the whole care team, echoing providers' comments about the benefits. But some of their examples also highlighted the negative impact one team member can have. Lona talked about how grateful she is to have found medical providers who are kind, knowledgeable, and unbiased. But she made the point that if someone else on the team is rude, condescending, or judgmental, the patient still has to endure that. She suggested that supervisors observe their staff's interactions with patients and provide training when needed. She says, "Even if it's fake at that moment, be empathetic… Try to have a little more compassion."

Care navigator

If you work in a setting that doesn't have support services, but does have critical follow-up, high care coordination needs, or patients with multiple barriers, there's one role I would strongly suggest you consider adding to your practice: A care navigator. Sometimes called a care coordinator or clinical case manager, these roles are often filled by medical social workers or nurses who have special knowledge and skill in helping patients navigate the health system. In some outpatient settings, community health workers may fill this role, supporting patients in following their care plan and connecting them to local resources.

Adding this role can literally be a lifesaver for patients. A navigator can check in with patients who have chronic conditions or challenges with adherence, help find resources to reduce barriers, and ensure the patient is clear on the treatment plan and any referrals or follow-up needed. Navigators more than pay for themselves with improved outcomes, saved provider time, reduced no-shows, etc. If you're in a small practice and don't have the volume, consider sharing this role between multiple practices. There's also a growing business of independent contractors who provide this service on a per diem basis for patients or clinics.

Many Medicare and Medicaid managed care plans, and some commercial insurances, now have some version of this for their complex or chronic care patients. Lona discussed the positive experience she had with a care navigator through her previous insurance plan; when any need came up that impacted her medical care, Lona says, "She was on it." If you can't have a care navigator or case manager of your own, it's worth the time to check with the patient's payer and see if this is available. In my conversations with insurance administrators, they say these programs are sometimes underutilized by patients who could benefit from them.

Space and messaging

When I was an undergrad, I did an internship at a small outpatient mental health practice. The practice was located in a house that had been converted into offices in an older, lower-income part of town. It was furnished with solid, practical furniture that was comfortable and meant to last. It was clean and welcoming, but certainly not fancy.

While I was interning there, a new building opened up near downtown. This was a beautiful high-rise – the loveliest building I had ever seen. It was tall with aesthetic angles and expansive surfaces of reflective glass that changed color with the sun. A friend and I went in to explore it one day. The atrium lobby was just as elegant. High ceilings, rich interior décor, well-kept live foliage everywhere. Lots of finely dressed people walking around in suits and heels. When we peeked around to see what businesses had leased space there, I was shocked to see some of the suites advertising mental health practices. My professional experiences up to that point had only been with the state CPS and foster care system and the internship in the older part of town. The contrast in physical space was striking. And the demographics the two practices were aiming for were very apparent.

The point I'm making isn't that we shouldn't work in a beautiful space in a nice part of town. Lower socioeconomic patients deserve to receive care in beautiful surroundings just as higher-SES patients do. The point is to develop awareness of what you're messaging to patients.

Creative solutions

Once we've identified barriers for the patient, we may need to be creative in finding solutions. As Dr. Whittier put it, "Especially in underserved communities, because they don't have the resources… There's a lot of creativity on the ground." This is a chance to think outside of standard practice – but within ethical and professional boundaries, of course. A few examples follow to give you an idea of what I mean.

Connecting with the patient's family members or advocates can open new avenues for effective treatment. Dr. Whittier shared a story about an elderly GYN patient who had some bleeding; when they did a biopsy they found endometrial cancer. The MA called the patient to schedule her to come in and discuss the results, but couldn't reach her for several attempts. When she finally got hold of her, the patient insisted she couldn't come because she didn't have transportation. Dr. Whittier called the patient herself, and the patient said the same thing. Dr. Whitter was aware that she had two sons, one of whom often brought her to appointments. She asked the patient if it was okay if she called her son to see about bringing her in. The patient agreed but had the wrong number for her son. After trying to reach him, Dr. Whittier called the patient again and asked if she could call her other son. She got the second son's number and was able to reach him and he brought the patient in.

Doing as much as you can during the visit or while the patient is present is also helpful; this can address time, transportation, and health literacy barriers. For example, rather than giving the patient a link to watch an informational video at home, have them watch it right then in the waiting room, or their inpatient room, or ER bed. If they have any questions or concerns, they can be addressed in real time. If the patient struggles to fill prescriptions because of cost, have a member of the team call a few pharmacies to find the cheapest cost for their prescription and then give the patient directions. Or take a few minutes while the patient is present to look online together to find which specialist is closest to their house that takes their insurance.

Sometimes simple solutions make the biggest difference. For a patient with multiple medications and difficulty reading – or difficulty reading the small print on prescription bottles – take a sharpie and write a basic instruction on each of the bottle caps: "One pill - AM." Once we open our minds to find simple, creative solutions for patient barriers, we can save ourselves and our patients time, frustration, and risk.

What if it's too much?

What if a patient's needs are just too much? You've recognized the significant social determinants of health that are impacting the patient. You've done your best to help them address those barriers, but it's gone beyond the resources you have available. You – and the patient – are feeling stuck. In this case, consider a referral. Many communities have community health centers (CHCs) and federally qualified health centers (FQHCs). These practices offer more wrap-around care than other practices are able. If you've decided you need to refer a patient, Dr. Larsen recommends simply telling the patient that you feel another clinic or healthcare team will be able to support their needs in ways that you can't. "Be honest," she says, "Don't make up stories about why you're not going to care for them anymore. Be honest with yourself."

Reflection

1) What prevents you from asking patients about the impact of their income, education, or occupation on their healthcare? Time? Discomfort? Not knowing how to ask, or not knowing what to do with the information once you have it?

2) Think about your standard phrasing and non-verbal communication during exams or appointments. Does it invite patients to express concerns and barriers? Or does it imply you'd prefer that they not?

3) Walk through your practice location as a patient would and see it with an objective eye. What does the décor say? What do the magazines in the lobby convey about who's supposed to be sitting there? Can you make subtle changes to ensure everyone walking in feels welcome?

CHAPTER 11
Internal Strategies

The only way to be there with the person in front of you is to be there with yourself first: 'I'm not hearing them through the lens of a provider but I'm hearing them first through the lens of being another human being.'

- DARLENE K.

When we discover our own biases or limitations, we like to attribute them to a lot of different factors: our upbringing, a formative experience we had, lack of exposure to the group in question… and these can all be true. But the fact is, there's another factor that is universal. It doesn't just apply to the majority culture, or to people with specific experiences (or lack thereof). We carry it around with us and it takes great effort to overcome it; I doubt anyone is ever able to overcome it fully. That factor is what some neuroscientists call the "3-pound universe": our brain. Or more specifically, the way our brain seems hard-wired to view the world and other people. In this next section, we jump into this inner world with strategies that will hopefully stretch your perception and challenge your thinking.

Increase awareness

The first – and most foundational – strategy is what this book has been focused on up to this point: Increasing our awareness. Does this contradict what I said earlier about insight being a booby prize? Insight and awareness may not be sufficient for change to occur, but sometimes they're still necessary.

If you've read this book from the beginning and didn't jump ahead, then you're already ahead of the game on this one. The goal is to become aware of your own assumptions, biases, automatic thoughts, and emotional reactions that are related to someone's socioeconomic status. The reflective questions I included throughout the book are meant to help you on that journey. If you've found these helpful, feel free to email me directly at my contact information in the back of the book; I'm happy to send you a complete list of questions in a format that can be shared with colleagues or students.

Cognitive stretches

SES flex

The next time a patient is sitting in your exam room with all the classic trappings of someone with a low SES, conduct a little thought experiment: Change their SES. Imagine that this person is actually a rich, eccentric genius. They have three post-graduate degrees; they personally hold patents to no less than a hundred cutting-edge tech advancements that are running in your devices at this very moment. They own that big house on the hill you've always admired. But they hate shopping for new clothes; they like to wear their favorites until they're so old they're falling off. They overslept this morning, rushing out of the house without showering or even combing their hair. Oh, and they hate dentists.

Now observe yourself: What does this experiment do to your approach to the patient? Your communication with them? The interventions you recommend?

Alternative explanations

As we've discussed, it's easy to fall into automatic assumptions about why people do the things they do. Sometimes these are informed by the narratives we've been exposed to; sometimes by the Self-Serving Bias; sometimes by the impact their behavior has on us, for better or worse.

One strategy I particularly like is to generate hypothetical alternative explanations for someone's behavior. For example, if a patient has no-showed for their appointment – and it's not the first time – it's easy for automatic assumptions and narratives about irresponsibility, disorganization, not making their health a priority, etc., to pop up. Instead of just accepting these automatic thoughts, take a moment to generate other possible explanations. Use your imagination.

For example, imagine that this patient was very invested in seeing you today. They got up early and were ready to go in plenty of time. Then, at the last minute, the babysitter called and cancelled. They tried their back-up options for childcare but couldn't find any. The appointment is important to them, so rather than cancelling they decide they'll just have to bring the kids with them. They rush to get the kids ready as quickly as they can and run everyone down the street to the bus stop or train station, only to find they've just missed it. The next one won't arrive for another 30 minutes. They wait and then hurry into your office. But it's too late; they're now 20 minutes late for the appointment and have to reschedule.

The point isn't whether this hypothetical scenario you've created is true or not. The point is breaking out of automatic assumptions that reinforce negative narratives and stereotypes. Purposefully creating and envisioning reasons that don't play into our implicit biases can be a powerful way to combat them.

Hypothesize reality

The title of this section sounds a bit odd, doesn't it? What do I mean by hypothesizing reality? Imagine this: A patient comes in and says the itchy rash on their hands started a week ago and they don't know where it came from. Unless this person has a history of being a poor historian or fabricating medical conditions, you accept this statement as real and accurate. This acceptance of the objective reality of a patient's statement doesn't always apply to lower SES patients, however. When a low SES patient says they don't have time to add something as simple as a ten-minute walk to their daily routine, or their life is too busy to check their blood sugar consistently, or they can't take time off work to get their lab work done… Why do we question the accuracy of this perception?

Instead, hypothesize that their perception and reporting of the situation is 100% real and true. Accepting this as the reality then allows us to be creative about finding a way around those barriers.

Find contradictory evidence

Once you've identified some of your specific stereotypes, assumptions, and biases, it's time to start actively combatting them. I mentioned above the Self-Serving Bias in Attribution: the tendency to attribute our own poor behavior to something external and our positive behavior to something internal, but to attribute the opposite for other people. There's another cognitive tendency that likewise makes it hard to change our perceptions: Confirmation Bias.

Our brains are hard-wired to seek out – and believe – information that confirms our existing beliefs and pre-conceptions, and at the same time to ignore, dismiss, or forget information that refutes it. If I believe my co-worker is lazy, I'm going to notice and remember the times I saw them coming to work late or scrolling on their phone when they should have been doing their job. I'm much less likely to notice – and more likely to forget or dismiss if I do notice – the times when they stayed late to finish something, worked through lunch, or got something done faster and better than the other employees.

It's easy to see how this applies to socioeconomic biases. Perhaps we have an implicit belief that lower-income parents are not as good at parenting. Imagine the negative stereotype: the mom in the grocery store with "too many" kids trailing behind. The kids are running around, being disruptive and disrespectful, the mom is yelling at them and dropping f-bombs. If this is a stereotypical category we have in our head: "Low SES Bad Mom," then any time we see a version of this played out, our brain will home in and magically transport that image right into that category. The more times it happens, the stronger the category becomes.

The way to combat Confirmation Bias is to actively attend to any examples we come across that provide the opposite evidence. Look for times when we see a family that seems to fit the stereotype, but then doesn't: The parent is managing the kids beautifully, the kids are well-behaved, and she addresses their misbehavior like a parenting pro. Maybe she's even taking the opportunity to teach them math, or budgeting, or nutrition using the items they're buying.

When we see examples that contradict our stereotype, the trick is to focus on them specifically and purposefully. Surreptitiously observe them (for as long as you can without being creepy). Then think about what you observed. Compare it to the stereotypical category and note how it differs. After the moment has passed, make a point of reflecting on it several times. If appropriate, share it with someone. This purposeful effort is what fights Confirmation Bias and allows more space within that category for a breadth of experiences and realities to exist.

Relate your own experience

Think back to one of the most stressful periods of your life. A time when whatever was going on felt all-consuming. You were distracted, you couldn't concentrate, your mind either froze or raced, your emotions were completely overwhelming. Maybe it lasted a day, maybe it lasted for months. This is what it's like to live with chronic financial insecurity: Fear of losing jobs, losing housing, unpaid bills, wondering whether you'll have enough food to eat, living in an unsafe area because you can't afford anywhere else, dread of an unexpected expense that will turn a tenuous situation into a full-blown crisis. That level of stress makes managing life tasks – and medical needs – much harder. Remembering the times when we've experienced overwhelming stress helps us have understanding and empathy for what it's like for our patients.

Set your mindset

Several providers I interviewed mentioned the importance of the mindset we bring into the room with us. Are we rushed? Annoyed? Are our implicit biases running unchecked?

The fact is, both the patient and care team are bringing more into their interaction than is visible. The care team member may be struggling with burnout, time pressure, or a sense of powerlessness. In addition, if there's work-related stress with co-workers, a supervisor, or new policies or procedures, these may be having a direct impact on what's happening in their workday.

The patient may be bringing embarrassment, anxiety about the issue they're seeking care for, or an expectation of judgment from their provider. As Darlene explained, "They [medical professionals] have to understand that when you've either lived your whole life in a lower socioeconomic status or you've hit it because your health has been demolished in some way, we are looking for proof that we're alone, that we're invisible, that nobody cares…"

I recommend building a new practice into your day that I'll call "The 3 Breaths." Right before you walk into the next exam room, stop outside the door, and take three breaths. With the first exhale, blow out whatever just happened with the last patient, the boss, your ex-spouse… whatever is keeping you from approaching that next patient with the right mindset. With the second exhale, consciously drop your shoulders and relax the muscles in your face. With the final exhale, set your mind to be open and compassionate.

Taking this moment not only helps move us into the right mental space to approach the patient, but it also helps the patient receive us in the right space to work collaboratively, advocate for themselves, and have an honest conversation. Dr. Whittier asserted, "You cannot walk in a room with assumptions about anyone. That is very dangerous, and I think it's very harmful. Very harmful. Walking in with compassion, conserving their dignity and open to hear their story. Without assuming you know their story."

It'll take some purposeful practice to make this a habit. Here's how to do it:

First, practice the 3 breaths at times when you're not at work. Do it in your car sitting at a stoplight, while you're doing the dishes, watching TV, etc. A non-rushed, non-stressed time.

Next, translate it to the work setting. Practice it at work, but outside of direct patient care. Try it while you're working on documentation, heading to lunch, etc.

Then, build the habit. Before each patient, do the 3 breaths. You'll need to be diligent about it at first. Put a colored sticky note on the outside of the exam room doors or some other visual cue that catches your attention long enough to stop and practice.

You may need to let the other members of your care team know what you're doing, or you can expect a lot of, "Are you alright?" when they see you pausing to breathe before every patient encounter.

Over time, as you internalize the steps, the three breaths can be consolidated into one, with the same benefits.

Us vs Them

When you're working with a patient who seems worlds away from where you are in life, make an effort to note the similarities as well as the differences. Consider how it could have been possible for you to end up in the same life situation as your patient. I'll use myself as an example of what I mean: Of the siblings I grew up with, I am the most "successful" by the mainstream standards we use in our culture. I have a college education; I'm financially stable; I've never been homeless; I haven't struggled with debilitating mental illness or substance use disorders; I've spent my adulthood gainfully employed. Suffice to say, this has not been the life experience of most of my siblings.

As nice as it would feel to give myself credit for this difference between us – it's because I was smarter, worked harder, made better choices, blah, blah, blah – I know that much of it was just plain old dumb luck. A biological roll of the dice where I rolled sevens and elevens and they got snake eyes.

The factors that lead us down one path or another are complex and interwoven. Yes, I probably did make some smart choices along the way. And yes, I definitely worked hard. But I also got the lucky biology of a brain that isn't particularly impulsive, doesn't especially enjoy drugs and alcohol, and has a boringly stable temperament. That wasn't my doing – trust me, I gave my brain plenty of opportunities to change its mind when I was young. But having a lot of the same risk factors for substance use, mental illness, and an unstable life that my siblings did – including my own behaviors and choices – I was the one who came out without those challenges.

For most of us, our life path hasn't been perfectly linear and predictable. Where we end up is influenced by more factors than we're even aware of. Family dynamics, genetics and epigenetics, early trauma and early support, influential relationships... all these and many more play a role. Think back on your life and consider the myriad of tiny differences that could have resulted in your present circumstances resembling those of your lower SES patients.

Reflection

1) What is the first automatic emotion, word, image, or assumption that comes into your head when your low SES patient:

   a. Brings their 3 young children into the exam room with them

   b. Smells like they haven't showered in two weeks

   c. Hasn't completed the lab work you already ordered twice

2) What is the first automatic emotion, word, image, or assumption that comes into your head when your *high* SES patient:

   a. Brings their 3 young children into the exam room with them

   b. Smells like they haven't showered in two weeks

   c. Hasn't completed the lab work you already ordered twice

CHAPTER 12
The Good Stuff

You have a lot of power to do good.

– Ivy Spadone, PA-C

Patient care is hard. It's hard regardless of the socioeconomic status of our patients. When you add a lack of basic resources into the mix, it can be downright demoralizing. But as much harder as it is to effectively treat our vulnerable patients, it's also that much more rewarding.

I asked providers what they enjoyed most in their work with lower SES patients. They talked about the amazing impact that small health changes can make. They talked about the powerful connection with their patients. They talked about being a positive force in the lives of people who have so much stacked against them.

If you work in healthcare in any capacity, you're already making a difference in people's lives. The ideas I've presented are simply opportunities to elevate your work for the patients who need it most. Will the recommendations in this book fix the fundamental problems in our healthcare system? Probably not. But they can have a profound impact on the patient sitting in front of you.

The patients I interviewed told story after story of small moments that made a big difference: a physician who looked them in the eye and took their concerns seriously; a kind smile and supportive comment from the person who checked them in; a treatment plan that was adjusted slightly so the patient could be successful, despite their limitations. For the care team, these moments were just a normal part of a normal day. But for the patient, it made a big enough impression to remember and share with me months or years later.

I'm a firm believer in the cumulative power of little efforts. Small changes in your practice, in your understanding of SES, and in face-to-face moments with individual patients can have a larger impact than you think:

A patient has a positive experience with you during their encounter and tells their neighbor. That neighbor hasn't sought medical care in years but is now willing to give it a try. They have a good experience and tell their cousin, who tells their friend… and the patient narrative begins to change.

A patient feels seen and understood by the diabetes educator and begins to take their management seriously. They get their blood sugar under control. Their kids see that they aren't being admitted to the hospital anymore and learn that they have the power to impact their own health. Those kids later model that self-efficacy for their children, who model it for their children.

The "ripple effect" is real. It's not as dramatic as broad, sweeping changes. But conscientious care, informed by our understanding of socioeconomic barriers and strategies to address them, can be even more powerful. Each small modification we make in our practice has a direct impact on someone's life. And that impact generates ripples out to other lives. If you could trace all the people your work benefits – both directly and indirectly – you'd see a vast network of ever-expanding positive change, moving across times and places you never could have imagined.

Chad's story exemplifies the power that healthcare professionals have. You'll recall that earlier in Chad's life he was enjoying a high socioeconomic lifestyle, living at Lake Tahoe, and running a successful art gallery. His fall was dramatic; he lost everything. But that's not the end of his story. Today, Chad works at the same health center that took care of him when he was at his lowest. He got back on his feet and became a Certified Peer Recovery Support Specialist: a professional who's in recovery from their own lived experience with addiction, mental health struggles, or homelessness and is trained to assist people in the same situation. Chad is now an integral part of the care team, making a real difference in people's lives.

Chad worked incredibly hard to get where he is. But he also credits the professionals who helped him. He insists we can't underestimate the power that we have: "These things change the trajectory of someone's life… I've been on both sides of the fence where things were really good, and things were really bad, and now the trajectory is returning to a better place. And my healthcare providers had so much to do with it."

Final reflection

1) Recall a specific patient whose life you impacted. Now imagine some of the ways that positive impact may have "rippled out" to their friends, family, or community.

2) Of all the information and concepts presented in this book, reflect on one thing you most want to remember a year from now.

ACKNOWLEDGMENTS

Many thanks to all the people who encouraged me, inspired me, and contributed to the creation of this book: my excellent accountability partner, Gene Killian; Matt Rudnitsky and Platypus Publishing; the people who generously contributed their insights and expertise: Chad J, Darlene K, Feather C, Jenna W, Lona S, Alexandra Macrenaris, Faith Whittier, Ivy Spadone, Jose Cucalon Calderon, Steve Shane, and Trudy Larson; my beta readers: Anne Wallace, Coral Paris, Jennifer Bowler, Judy Primm-Shimahara, Laura Drucker, Malynda Tushbant, Mary Duffy, Nancy Podewils-Baba, and Nicole Jacobs; the staff and leadership of Northern Nevada HOPES, who do amazing work and helped me decide on the title for this book; and finally, my two wonderful children, who inspire me to keep working to make the world a better place.

APPENDIX A
Social Determinants of Health: Patient Questionnaires

The American Academy of Family Physicians Social Needs Screening Tool
  https://aafp.org/dam/AAFP/documents/patient_care/everyone_project/patient-short-print.pdf

The Protocol for Responding to and Accessing Patients' Assets, Risks, and Experiences
  (PRAPARE). http://nachc.org/research-and-data/prapare/toolkit/

Accountable Health Communities Health-Related Social Needs Screening Tool (AHC-HRSN). https://www.cms.gov/priorities/innovation/files/worksheets/ahcm-screeningtool.pdf/

APPENDIX B
Social Determinants of Health: Resources for Patients

These websites provide links to a variety of community resources, agencies, and social services:
  http://www.211.org or call 211
  https://www.findhelp.org
  https://www.CatholicCharitiesUSA.org

Housing and food assistance:
  Supplemental Nutrition Assistance Program: http://www.fns.usda.gov/snap
  Special Supplemental Nutrition Program for Women, Infants, and Children (WIC): http://www.fns.usda.gov/wic
  Public Housing and Voucher Program: http://www.hud.gov/topics/rental_assistance

Most communities also have the following local supports available:
  Food banks
  Discount programs for public transportation
  Rotary Clubs
  Support programs through local churches

APPENDIX C
Motivational Interviewing Resources

Motivational Interviewing: Helping People Change and Grow, Fourth Edition, by Stephen Rollnick and William R. Miller (2023) Motivational Interviewing: Helping People Change and Grow (Applications of Motivational Interviewing Series): 9781462552795: Medicine & Health Science Books @ Amazon.com

Motivational Interviewing in Healthcare: Helping Patients Change Behavior, Second Edition, by Stephen Rollnick, William R. Miller, and Christopher C. Butler (2022) Amazon.com: Motivational Interviewing in Health Care: Helping Patients Change Behavior (Applications of Motivational Interviewing Series): 9781462550371: Rollnick, Stephen, Miller, William R., Butler, Christopher C.: Books

Building Motivational Interviewing Skills: A Practitioner Workbook, Second Edition, by David B. Rosengren (2017) Building Motivational Interviewing Skills: A Practitioner Workbook (Applications of Motivational Interviewing Series): 9781462532063: Medicine & Health Science Books @ Amazon.com

Motivational Interviewing in Nutrition and Fitness, by Dawn Clifford and Laura Curtis (2015) Motivational Interviewing in Nutrition and Fitness (Applications of Motivational Interviewing Series): 9781462524181: Medicine & Health Science Books @ Amazon.com

Motivational Interviewing Network of Trainers (MINT), https://motivationalinterviewing.org/

Certificate of Intensive Training in Motivational Interviewing, UMass Chan Medical School, https://www.umassmed.edu/cipc/continuing-education/MotivationalInterviewing/

Each healthcare profession has training in MI specific to their role, and there are resources focused on different topics, such as substance use, diabetes, or heart disease. In addition, there are many, many YouTube videos with introductions to the concepts of MI and videotaped role plays or patient interactions using an MI approach.

REFERENCES

1. Shrider EA, Creamer J. *Poverty in the United States: 2022.* United States Census Bureau. September 12, 2023. Accessed March 16, 2024. https://www.census.gov/library/publications/2023/demo/p60-280.html

2. U.S. Bureau of Labor Statistics. Standard Occupational Classification. Accessed November 11, 2023. https://www.bls.gov/soc/

3. Adler NE, Epel ES, Castellazzo G, Ickovics JR. Relationship of subjective and objective social status with psychological and physiological functioning: preliminary data in healthy white women. *Health Psychol.* 2000 Nov;19(6):586-92. doi: 10.1037//0278-6133.19.6.586

4. Jones EJ, Marsland AL, Kraynak TE, Votruba-Drzal E, Gianaros PJ. Subjective Social Status and Longitudinal Changes in Systemic Inflammation. *Ann Behav Med.* 2023 Oct 16;57(11):951-964. doi: 10.1093/abm/kaad044

5. Garza JR, Glenn BA, Mistry RS, Ponce NA, Zimmerman FJ. Subjective Social Status and Self-Reported Health Among US-born and Immigrant Latinos. *J Immigr Minor Health.* 2017 Feb;19(1):108-119. doi: 10.1007/s10903-016-0346-x

6. Goodman E, Adler NE, Daniels SR, Morrison JA, Slap GB, Dolan LM. Impact of objective and subjective social status on obesity in a

biracial cohort of adolescents. *Obes Res.* 2003 Aug;11(8):1018-26. doi: 10.1038/oby.2003.140

7. Singh-Manoux A, Adler NE, Marmot MG. Subjective social status: its determinants and its association with measures of ill-health in the Whitehall II study. *Soc Sci Med.* 2003 Mar;56(6):1321-33. doi: 10.1016/s0277-9536(02)00131-4

8. Cohen S, Alper CM, Doyle WJ, Adler N, Treanor JJ, Turner RB. Objective and subjective socioeconomic status and susceptibility to the common cold. *Health Psychol.* 2008 Mar;27(2):268-74. doi: 10.1037/0278-6133.27.2.268

9. Cundiff JM, Matthews KA. Is subjective social status a unique correlate of physical health? A meta-analysis. *Health Psychol.* 2017 Dec;36(12):1109-1125. doi: 10.1037/hea0000534

10. Guralnik JM, Land KC, Blazer D, Fillenbaum GG, & Branch LG. (1993). Educational Status and Active Life Expectancy among Older Blacks and Whites. *N Engl J Med.* 1993;329(2):110–116. https://doi.org/10.1056/NEJM199307083290208

11. Barr, DA. *Health Disparities in the United States: Social Class, Race, Ethnicity, and the Social Determinants of Health.* 3rd edition. Johns Hopkins University Press. 2019.

12. World Health Organization. Social Determinants of Health. Accessed November 11. 2023. https://www.who.int/health-topics/social-determinants-of-health#tab=tab_1

13. Mateyka, PJ, Yoo, J. *Share of Income Needed to Pay Rent Increased the Most for Low-Income Households from 2019-2021.* United States Census Bureau. Revised February 28,2023. Accessed March 16, 2024. https://www.census.gov/library/stories/2023/03/low-income-renters-spent-larger-share-of-income-on-rent.html

14. Besser LM, Rodriguez DA, McDonald N, Kukull WA, Fitzpatrick AL, Rapp SR, Seeman T. Neighborhood built environment and cognition in non-demented older adults: The Multi-Ethnic Study of

Atherosclerosis. *Soc Sci Med.* 2018 Mar;200:27-35. doi: 10.1016/j.socscimed.2018.01.007

15. Nobel L, Jesdale WM, Tjia J, Waring ME, Parish DC, Ash AS, Kiefe CI, Allison JJ. Neighborhood Socioeconomic Status Predicts Health After Hospitalization for Acute Coronary Syndromes: Findings From TRACE-CORE (Transitions, Risks, and Actions in Coronary Events-Center for Outcomes Research and Education). *Med Care.* 2017 Dec;55(12):1008-1016. doi: 10.1097/MLR.0000000000000819

16. Robinette JW, Charles ST, Gruenewald TL. Neighborhood cohesion, neighborhood disorder, and cardiometabolic risk. *Soc Sci Med.* 2018 Feb;198:70-76. doi: 10.1016/j.socscimed.2017.12.025

17. Scott SB, Munoz E, Mogle JA, Gamaldo AA, Smyth JM, Almeida DM, Sliwinski MJ. Perceived neighborhood characteristics predict severity and emotional response to daily stressors. *Soc Sci Med.* 2018 Mar;200:262-270. doi: 10.1016/j.socscimed.2017.11.010

18. Centers for Disease Control and Prevention. Violence Prevention: We Can Prevent Childhood Adversity. CDC. Published June 30, 2021. Accessed November 11, 2023. https://vetoviolence.cdc.gov/apps/aces-infographic/

19. Harvard University. Outsmarting Implicit Bias. Accessed September 10, 2023. https://outsmartingimplicitbias.org/

20. Jussim L, Thulin E, Fish J, Wright JD (contributors). *Articles Critical of the IAT and Implicit Bias.* Open Science Framework. Created July 10, 2020. Updated March 11, 2023. Accessed September 10, 2023. https://osf.io/74whk/

21. van Ryn M, Burke J. The effect of patient race and socio-economic status on physicians' perceptions of patients. *Soc Sci Med.* 2000 Mar;50(6):813-28. doi: 10.1016/s0277-9536(99)00338-x

22. Woo JK, Ghorayeb SH, Lee CK, Sangha H, Richter S. Effect of patient socioeconomic status on perceptions of first- and second-year medical students. *CMAJ.* 2004 Jun 22;170(13):1915-9. doi: 10.1503/cmaj.1031474

23. Brandão T, Campos L, de Ruddere L, Goubert L, Bernardes SF. Classism in Pain Care: The Role of Patient Socioeconomic Status on Nurses' Pain Assessment and Management Practices. *Pain Med.* 2019 Nov 1;20(11):2094-2105. doi: 10.1093/pm/pnz148

24. Lechtholz-Zey E, Bonney PA, Cardinal T, Mendoza J, Strickland BA, Pangal DJ, Giannotta S, Durham S, Zada G. Systematic Review of Racial, Socioeconomic, and Insurance Status Disparities in the Treatment of Pediatric Neurosurgical Diseases in the United States. *World Neurosurg.* 2022 Feb;158:65-83. doi: 10.1016/j.wneu.2021.10.150

25. Obialo CI, Ofili EO, Quarshie A, & Martin PC. Ultralate Referral and Presentation for Renal Replacement Therapy: Socioeconomic Implications. *Am J Kidney Dis*, 2005;46(5):881–886. https://doi.org/10.1053/j.ajkd.2005.08.003

26. Navaneethan SD, Aloudat S, & Singh S. A systematic review of patient and health system characteristics associated with late referral in chronic kidney disease. *BMC Nephrology*, 2008;9(1):3–3. https://doi.org/10.1186/1471-2369-9-3

27. Gad KT, Johansen C, Duun-Henriksen AK, Krøyer A, Olsen MH, Lassen U, Mau-Sørensen M, & Oksberg Dalton S. Socioeconomic Differences in Referral to Phase I Cancer Clinical Trials: A Danish Matched Cancer Case-Control Study. *J of Clin Oncology*, 2019;37(13), 1111–1119. https://doi.org/10.1200/JCO.18.01983

28. Dehlendorf C, Ruskin R, Grumbach K, Vittinghoff E, Bibbins-Domingo K, Schillinger D, Steinauer J. Recommendations for intrauterine contraception: a randomized trial of the effects of patients' race/ethnicity and socioeconomic status. *Am J Obstet Gynecol.* 2010 Oct;203(4):319.e1-8. doi: 10.1016/j.ajog.2010.05.009

29. Harrison DD, Cooke CW. An elucidation of factors influencing physicians' willingness to perform elective female sterilization. *Obstet Gynecol.* 1988 Oct;72(4):565-70. PMID: 3419736.

30. Weiner SS, Weiser SR, Carragee EJ, Nordin M. Managing nonspecific low back pain: do nonclinical patient characteristics matter? *Spine* (Phila Pa 1976). 2011 Nov 1;36(23):1987-94. doi: 10.1097/BRS.0b013e3181fee8ef

31. Dumesnil H, Cortaredona S, Verdoux H, Sebbah R, Paraponaris A, & Verger P. General Practitioners' Choices and Their Determinants When Starting Treatment for Major Depression: A Cross Sectional, Randomized Case-Vignette Survey. *PloS One*, 2012;7(12), e52429–e52429. https://doi.org/10.1371/journal.pone.0052429

32. Shapiro N, Wachtel EV, Bailey SM, Espiritu MM. Implicit Physician Biases in Periviability Counseling. *J Pediatr.* 2018 Jun;197:109-115.e1. doi: 10.1016/j.jpeds.2018.01.070

33. Addala A, Hanes S, Naranjo D, Maahs DM, Hood KK. Provider Implicit Bias Impacts Pediatric Type 1 Diabetes Technology Recommendations in the United States: Findings from The Gatekeeper Study. *J Diabetes Sci Technol.* 2021 Sep;15(5):1027-1033. doi: 10.1177/19322968211006476

34. Shackelton RJ, Marceau LD, Link CL, McKinlay JB. The intended and unintended consequences of clinical guidelines. *J Eval Clin Pract.* 2009 Dec;15(6):1035-42. doi: 10.1111/j.1365-2753.2009.01201.x

35. Williams RL, Romney C, Kano M, Wright R, Skipper B, Getrich CM, Sussman AL, Zyzanski SJ. Racial, gender, and socioeconomic status bias in senior medical student clinical decision-making: a national survey. *J Gen Intern Med.* 2015 Jun;30(6):758-67. doi: 10.1007/s11606-014-3168-3

36. Denberg T. Patient race and outcome preferences as predictors of urologists' treatment recommendations and referral patterns in early-stage prostate cancer. *Sci Tech Aerosp Rep*, 2006;44(18).

37. Gopaul R, Waller RA, Kalayanamitra R, Rucker G, Foy A. Evaluation of Provider Assessment of Clinical History When Using the HEART

Score. *Open Access Emerg Med.* 2022 Aug 4;14:421-428. doi: 10.2147/OAEM.S371502

38. Schnitzer PK. "THEY DON'T COME IN!": Stories Told, Lessons Taught About Poor Families in Therapy. *Am J Orthopsych*, 1996;66(4), 572–582. https://doi.org/10.1037/h0080206

39. Schmidt, E. Reading the Numbers: 130 Million American Adults Have Low Literacy Skills, but Funding Differs Drastically by State. APM Research Lab. March 16, 2022. Accessed November 15, 2023. https://www.apmresearchlab.org/10x-adult-literacy#:~:text=by%20EMILY%20SCHMIDT%20%7C%20March%2016%2C%202022&text=This%20means%20more%20than%20half,of%20a%20sixth%2Dgrade%20level.

40. Rothwell, J. Assessing the Economic Gains of Eradicting Illiteracy Nationally and Regionally in the United States. Barbara Bush Foundation for Family Literacy. Published September 8, 2020. Accessed November 15, 2023. https://www.barbarabush.org/wp-content/uploads/2020/09/BBFoundation_GainsFromEradicatingIlliteracy_9_8.pdf

41. Healthy People 2030. Health Literacy in Healthy People 2030. Office of Disease Prevention and Health Promotion, Office of the Assistant Secretary for Health. https://health.gov/healthypeople/priority-areas/health-literacy-healthy-people-2030. Accessed November 15,2023.

42. Centers for Disease Control and Prevention. Health Literacy. Reviewed February 22, 2024. Accessed March 16, 2024. https://www.cdc.gov/healthliteracy/index.html

43. Willems S, De Maesschalck S, Deveugele M, Derese A, De Maeseneer J. Socio-economic status of the patient and doctor-patient communication: does it make a difference? *Patient Educ Couns.* 2005 Feb;56(2):139-46. doi: 10.1016/j.pec.2004.02.011

44. Malle BF. The Actor-Observer Asymmetry in Attribution: A (Surprising) Meta-Analysis. *Psychol Bull.* 2006;*132*(6), 895–919. https://doi.org/10.1037/0033-2909.132.6.895

CONTACT THE AUTHOR

Kristen Davis-Coelho, PhD | LinkedIn

kristendavis-coelho@outlook.com

Made in the USA
Las Vegas, NV
21 August 2024